THE SHARPBRAINS GUIDE TO BRAIN FITNESS

New and Expanded Second Edition

How to Optimize Brain Health
and Performance at Any Age

Alvaro Fernandez and Elkhonon Goldberg, PhD
With Pascale Michelon, PhD

Praise

for The SharpBrains Guide to Brain Fitness (first edition)

"One of those books you cannot ignore. Insightful, to the point, actionable. A book for leaders, innovators, thought provokers and everyone who wants to act and live smarter and healthier, based on latest neuroscience."

—**Dr. Tobias Kiefer**, Director Global Learning & Development, Booz & Company

"An essential reference on the field of brain fitness, neuroplasticity and cognitive health"

—**Walter Jessen,** PhD, founder and editor, Highlight Health

"Recognized by AARP as one of the best and most comprehensive source of information, this book manages to remain open minded yet adequately critical at the same—a good model for all sharp minds to follow and benefit from."

—**Dr. Peter Whitehouse,** Professor of Neurology at Case Western Reserve University

"A much-needed resource to help us better understand our brains and minds and how to nourish them through life."

—**Susan E. Hoffman,** Director, Osher Lifelong Learning Institute at UC Berkeley

"…the best overview I've seen of neuroscience implications for personal development and professional effectiveness"

—**Ed Batista,** Leadership Coach at the Stanford Graduate School of Business

"Kudos for an excellent resource! This book is full of top notch information and practical tips, and helps separate hype from hope in the brain health arena."

—**Elizabeth Edgerly,** Ph.D., Chief Program Officer, Alzheimer's Association

"The SharpBrains Guide To Brain Fitness reminds of us all why books (and not just googling a topic) can be well worth your time and money. Two Stethoscopes Up — check it out."

—**Dr. Jan Gurley,** Internist Physician and Robert Wood Johnson Fellow

"This book provides a very valuable service to a wide community interested in learning and brain topics."

—**Michael Posner,** Emeritus Professor of Neuroscience at the University of Oregon

"Finally, an insightful and complete overview of the science, products and trends to debunk old myths and help us all maintain our brains in top shape. A must-read"

—**Gloria Cavanaugh,** former President of the American Society on Aging

"A masterful guide to the brain training revolution. Promises to stimulate a much needed conversation that will nudge society to build a new brain fitness culture on solid, research-based, foundations."

—**P. Murali Doraiswamy MD,** Professor of Psychiatry, Duke University

"This is the only book that I know of that seamlessly integrates latest information about cognitive health across the lifespan. Very useful to anyone interested in the brain."

—**Arthur Kramer,** Professor of Psychology at University of Illinois

We dedicate this book
to your Unique Brain,
and your Unique Mind.

Table of contents

FOREWORD to the SECOND EDITION

Writing a foreword to this book against a tight deadline is a somewhat challenging task. As you will learn later in the book though, there is reason to believe that such mentally stimulating, novel activities are beneficial for keeping my brain sharp as I gain in wisdom – and in years. Like many people, I have noticed changes with aging since my younger adult years. And while we all wish for a magic pill, at least for the time being it is our behaviors, perhaps aided by technology, which can help us to age well physically, emotionally, and cognitively.

Indeed, novel information, communications, networking, and interface technologies are poised to transform the way we approach our lifelong health and well-being, including our very understanding of what it means to be healthy and well. As a program officer at the National Science Foundation, I have been witnessing multiple discoveries and advances stimulated by the NSF Smart Health and Wellbeing program that may bring substantial improvements to how we enhance health. With rapid progress in sensor, online and mobile technology, advances in the domain of Smart Health open a new world of possibility for the systematic monitoring and managing of long-term health outcomes, going far beyond the sporadic treatment of acute conditions. The notion of Smart Health places greater emphasis on the management of wellness, rather than healing illness; it acknowledges the role of home, family, and community as significant contributors to individual health and wellbeing; and it recognizes the central role of an individual's cognition in driving and maintaining healthy habits over time.

Alvaro Fernandez and I first met at a 2009 scientific symposium hosted by Arizona State University. I was there to give a talk about the promising potential in using computer games as a way to monitor and perhaps maintain cognition over time. Alvaro gave an insightful overview of the state of the science and marketplace for cognitive fitness. Mutual interests naturally led to a discussion after the talks and many exchanges thereafter. Since then, it has been my pleasure to participate in all three annual SharpBrains Virtual Summits held so far – they provide a unique opportunity to engage with colleagues at the forefront of the science, technology, and marketplace to support brain health and fitness across the lifespan. Our interactions included a September 2012 workshop on computer games, attention and well-being hosted by the White House Office of Science and Technology Policy and the National Science Foundation that brought together neuroscientists, cognitive scientists and game designers.

The need for such transdisciplinary collaboration has long been recognized by SharpBrains, the pioneering organization bringing you this book, which has for a number years been bringing together a community of neuroscientists and cognitive scientists working towards a better understanding of the human brain, technologists devising ways to scale platforms and solutions, as well practitioners and consumers looking for practical ways to make real changes in behavior and lifestyle to improve brain health and health overall. This book reflects this diversity, covering topics ranging from the complexity of the brain and its mechanisms to the significance of different types of scientific studies to practical aspects of exercising, nutrition, and training.

A resource like this book in your hands provides a great starting point: although there is no "final word" on this still nascent topic, an important transformation is underway that people need to be aware of and prepared for. This book is a great start for making sense of it all and for taking active steps towards smart health, at the individual level, and Smart Health, at the societal level. And while this book was written to be accessible to a wide audience, it remains a worthwhile and interesting read for experts as it provides a thoughtful and well-integrated summary of emerging findings and hypotheses. This combined value

– for the general and the expert reader – is in part achieved through the inclusion of candid interviews with top researchers and leaders in various relevant fields as well as succinct summaries and very clear structure and writing.

In short, no matter who you are, this is an important read. I hope you enjoy it.

Misha Pavel, PhD
Professor of Biomedical Engineering,
Oregon Health and Science University,
and Program Director for the
National Science Foundation's Smart
Health and Wellbeing Program.

FOREWORD to the FIRST EDITION

In the winter of 2007, as I was planning a new conference titled "Brain Health Across The Lifespan" with the Institute on Aging, I recognized the growing interest in the topic of brain fitness. This felt like a breath of fresh air. During my 30 years leading the American Society on Aging we focused heavily on the importance of lifelong learning and mental stimulation as an important component of healthy aging. Now that scientists know more about the lifelong neuroplasticity of our brains, and how our lifestyles, actions and thoughts influence the way our brains develop with age, newspapers, magazines, TV, and books, are enthusiastically covering the field of brain fitness and "brain training".

Widespread media coverage, though, combined with often contradictory or partial product claims, has contributed to confusion in the minds of some consumers and professionals as to how to navigate the growing array of options. Is doing one more crossword puzzle the best thing I can do for my brain? Or is it taking some vitamin supplements? Why are both physical and mental exercises so important, and complementary to each other? Why is managing stress as critical to cognitive health as, say, finding stimulating activities to do? What is the value of new "brain training games," and how can I evaluate and compare them?

For the Brain Health Across The Lifespan conference, I wanted to bring the best speakers and resources on the topic of brain fitness. Asking around dozens of colleagues, I came to hear the name Sharp-Brains over and over – peers mentioned how Dr. Elkhonon Goldberg and Alvaro Fernandez, co-founders of SharpBrains and co-authors of this guide, had been providing much-needed quality information about the growing field of brain fitness. This is why I invited Alvaro Fernandez to speak at our conference in 2008 and why I am honored to write this foreword.

Neuroscientist Dr. Elkhonon Goldberg and educator and executive Alvaro Fernandez have been working for years with dozens of scientists and experts to answer questions like those above. They founded SharpBrains, a market research company that covers the healthcare and educational applications of neuroscience, to provide information and services to its impressive roster of clients, including leading healthcare providers, insurance companies, universities, and more. I am pleased that they have now distilled much information and advice into this practical and thought-provoking guide.

I am sure that you will feel more enlightened, stimulated, and hopeful, after reading the eye-opening book you have in your hands – as I do.

Gloria Cavanaugh

Former President and CEO
of the American Society on Aging
and founding Board member
of the National Alliance for Caregiving

INTRODUCTION

Just ten years ago, it was still rare to see the word "brain" appear next to "fitness" or "training," or the word "cognitive" followed by "enhancement." Today, not a week goes by without a new media report or scientific announcement linking these words, a change reflective of the growing interest in optimizing brain function across the lifespan from both the scientific and medical community and the general population. Given the current reality of a complex, changing environment that places more lifelong cognitive demands on our brains than ever, and longer lives thanks to unprecedented gains in life span that have added more than 25 years to the U.S. life expectancy over the past century, this interest is quite timely.

2007 was a tipping point, as brain fitness burst into public awareness as a new aspiration. Significant scientific breakthroughs that year linked physical and mental exercise to lasting cognitive improvements. These discoveries were accompanied by a jump in media coverage throughout the year, ending with a PBS special titled "The Brain Fitness Program." Popular books on the topic made it to the *New York Times* Best Seller list, and, with Nintendo's Brain Age leading the way, dozens of products were introduced by companies hoping to capitalize on the growing buzz. From this early surge of interest things have developed steadily over the past six years, as brain fitness establishes a secure (yet not always well-informed) place in the popular imagination.

Making sense of the opportunity

As brain fitness goes mainstream, the accompanying proliferation of scientific findings, media coverage, and commercial claims has resulted in much noise and confusion. Research is rapidly evolving and often contradictory on the surface. News sources often report scientific findings or opinions out of context and carry educational messages of questionable relevance and quality. A variety of competing companies make fantastic claims about their products, often with little evidence or scientific backing. Knowing what to believe and whom to listen to can present a real challenge.

The story of two studies, published within weeks of each other in 2010, illustrates the importance of approaching this field with a discerning and cautious eye. The first study, sponsored by the BBC, was translated into hundreds of media stories with headlines like "Brain Training Doesn't Work." What the study actually showed is that gathering a collection of new and untested brain games in one website and asking people who happened to show up to play around for a total of just three to four hours over six weeks did not result in meaningful improvements in cognitive functioning. The study was criticized by scientists on a variety of grounds (including the surprising fact that all data collected from people over 60 had been excluded from the final analysis), but the mainstream story was conveniently clear-cut: "brain training" doesn't work. Case closed.

A short time later, a comprehensive study sponsored by the National Institute of Health (NIH) also made the news. This was a very extensive meta-analysis of the existing scientific literature aiming at a better understanding of the risk and protective factors for cognitive decline and Alzheimer's Disease (AD). This study, the most impressive of its kind as of March 2013, when this manuscript was finished, analyzed the results of 25 general reviews and 250 clinical studies using very rigorous methods. Upon its publication, the main message swiftly reported by the popular press was the unqualified verdict that "Nothing Can Prevent Alzheimer's Disease."

But the detailed analysis actually showed much more than that. A careful glance at the results reveals that several lifestyle factors clearly increased or decreased the risk of cognitive decline and AD. And, somewhat surprisingly, that cognitive training is one of the most clearly protective factors against cognitive decline. Which seems to contradict the findings from the BBC study, and presents us with a more complex state of affairs than we might have gathered just from the headlines. Since the media and most experts generally overlooked this part of the NIH analysis, most people were left unaware of these results. Instead, we are left with another cautionary illustration of the danger in relying on superficial or unreliable information in making decisions about something as important as the health and performance of your brain.

Preventing disease, optimizing health and performance, or both?

We believe that a primary reason for this confused state of affairs is the lack of a broad understanding of what "brain fitness" actually entails – what is brain fitness? Physical fitness refers to a state of physical well-being and functionality that allows us to carry out daily activities without too much physical difficulty. In the same way, true brain fitness refers to having the brain functionality – cognitive, emotional, executive – required to thrive in the environment we face each day – and those we are likely to face in years (and decades) to come.

From such a definition, it is clear that brain fitness matters for life, and throughout life. It is obvious that ignoring your body's health until your later years is unwise, and the same is true for your brain. Brain fitness, in other words, is not something to first start worrying about at age 60 or 70, and this is true for two reasons. First, optimizing brain functionality is a goal of interest at any age, as your brain's functioning impacts your ability to thrive and succeed at every point in life. For example, a survey conducted by SharpBrains in 2010 identified the ability to manage stressful situations, the concentration power to avoid distractions, and the ability to recognize and manage one's emotions as the brain functions recognized as most essential for thriving personally and professionally in the 21st century.

Second, growing evidence suggests beyond a reasonable doubt

that what we do at every single stage of life has an impact on brain fitness later in life. The way you treat your brain today can affect its health and ability years from now. Brain fitness priorities do change with age – and this is part of the challenge and the opportunity. Many children have special learning needs to deal with such as attention deficits or anxiety management issues. Better managing stress and regulating emotions may be priorities for younger adults. Memory performance may be a priority later in life.

We need to invest in a fuller, nuanced approach that is informed by emerging research and that emphasizes a more global view of brain fitness, not restricted to the prevention of dementia but encompassing the lifelong trajectory of one's brain health and performance. Our understanding of the brain is growing at an accelerating pace: In early 2013 President Obama announced plans for a decade-long effort to investigate the functioning and connectivity of the human brain, which will likely lead to significant advances in brain care. However, that is not to say that you should wait another ten years to be proactive and start taking care of your brain, just as it doesn't make much sense to wait a decade to buy a next generation car if you need to drive somewhere today.

The goal of this guide

When it comes to brain fitness behaviors and habits, you often hear people mention basic things like physical exercise and a good diet or repeat catchy phrases like "use it or lose it." This only scratches the surface. The profound implications of lifelong neurogenesis (creation of new neurons), lifelong neuroplasticity (rewiring the brain through experience) and cognitive reserve (delaying the onset of Alzheimer's Disease symptoms via mental stimulation) are too often trivialized in our society. It is not just about doing a few more crossword puzzles, eating a dozen blueberries with your breakfast cereal, or walking a bit more. A consequence of the brain's plasticity is that it may change with every experience, thought and emotion, from which it follows that you yourself have the potential power to change your brain with everything that you do, think, and feel. So brain fitness and optimization are about much more than crossword puzzles and blueberries; they are about cultivating a new mindset and mastering a new toolkit that allow us to appreciate and take full advantage of our brains' incredible properties.

Your brain is your most precious asset, and it is wise to invest in it accordingly. All too often, people devote plenty of time, energy, and attention to their bodies and to their financial portfolios without giving much thought to the very asset that will enable them to perform successfully in all those endeavors and enjoy the fruits of their labors. It does not make much sense to spend decades investing in a retirement fund to ensure financial security down the line without investing in the health and performance of the very brain you will need to enjoy that retirement.

Committing to work towards caring for and optimizing your brain is a good first step, but keeping track of the newest advances in the science, technology, and marketplace of brain fitness can be quite challenging and confusing. Fortunately, we did the work for you. This book is the result of seven years of extensive research, including interviews with more than a hundred scientists and professionals, surveys with thousands of consumers, reviews of hundreds of scientific publications, and three global conferences on the topic.

With this second edition of *The SharpBrains Guide to Brain Fitness*, we aspire to provide you with the information and understanding to make sound and personally relevant decisions about how to optimize your own brain health and performance – and perhaps to empower you to serve as an ambassador to spread the word in your community. Specifically we will strive to provide a basic understanding of brain function and demystify how the brain works, to discuss the lifestyle factors that matter most, and to review the pros and cons of a diverse assortment of research-based brain optimization methodologies, from mindfulness meditation programs to computerized cognitive training options.

We would like to emphasize that this Guide is intended for everyone with a brain who would like to learn how to maintain its health and strengthen its functioning. Our aim is not to provide a "prescription," but to enhance your ability to take charge of your own brain fitness in a mindful and conscious effort to build capacity and delay decline. In other words, we want to help you maximize your "cognitive and mental fitness trajectory," starting today and lasting for a lifetime. We hope it proves to be a worthy resource.

The SharpBrains Guide to Brain Fitness is organized into 9 chapters. Chapter 1 takes you inside the human brain and shows what neuroplasticity is and why it is at the core of brain fitness, and Chapter 2 provides the tools you need to better understand and apply new scientific findings. The following chapters describe the pillars of brain fitness – how to address the basics. Each pillar should be seen as a piece of the brain fitness puzzle: they are complementary and, according to the latest research, augment rather than substitute for one another. Chapter 3 provides evidence and guidelines regarding physical exercise and its impact on brain plasticity. Chapter 4 shows the role of balanced nutrition in brain health and explores the effects of health-related factors (such as diabetes, smoking, and obesity) on cognition. Chapter 5 focuses on cognitive engagement as a way to boost cognitive reserve and describes the lifelong factors that matter (i.e., education, occupation, and daily activities). Chapter 6 explores the impact of social engagement on brain functionality. Chapter 7 focuses on managing stress and building emotional resilience – an often overlooked factor. Chapter 8 goes beyond the lifestyle basics and focuses on how to cross-train the brain, discussing the techniques and tools that are gaining in popularity. Finally, Chapter 9 concludes the guide by summarizing what a reasonable person can do to navigate and apply all this knowledge and take control by becoming one's very own "brain fitness coach."

Each chapter also includes transcripts of interviews with prominent scientists conducted between 2006 and 2012. They provide in depth insights of the scientific topics covered, as well as open questions and doubts, straight from the minds of leading scientists. They complement, clarify, expand, and sometimes even challenge, each other and the main text. You can choose to read them as you go along, or to save them for later, as their primary insights have been incorporated into the main text.

Finally, please note that we do not prescribe or endorse any specific interventions. This guide aspires to offer independent, up-to-date information and analysis, and to empower you to exercise your unique brain and unique mind to optimize your brain health and performance now and in the future.

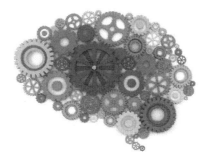

CHAPTER 1

START WITH THE BRAIN IN MIND

An aspiring clarinetist begins by getting a sense of the way the instrument's sounds are produced by the air he blows through it. A driver must be acquainted with various vehicle fundamentals, such as adding gas, accelerating, and reading the speedometer. It is no different with the brain. Maximizing your brain's health and performance begins with a basic understanding of how it works and how it evolves across the lifespan.

WHAT DOES THE BRAIN DO?

We are so used to the smooth functioning of our brains that we rarely pay much thought to what goes on "under the hood." Because most of what happens in the brain occurs below conscious awareness or control, the bulk of our actions throughout the day (walking, chewing food, discussing a book) seem natural and simple. It is quite easy to forget that our behaviors are actually the sophisticated productions of an incredibly complex organ.

To get a finer sense of how the brain's abilities – and limitations – impact everyday life, let's look at a few common situations and see what key (and often overlooked) brain functions are at play:

Working memory: You are talking with your financial adviser about your portfolio. He keeps throwing numbers and percentages at you. You try to figure out whether fund X (5% return, 5.75% service fees upfront, but no fee when you sell) is better for you than fund Y (4% return, no upfront fees, fees when you sell that decrease over the years). You try hard for a while to do some mental math and figure out the big picture; then your mental screen goes blank and you feel utterly confused. What functions were you using and why did they fail you? This is a perfect example of "working memory" overload. Working memory is the type of memory that allows us to both hold information in mind and work on it as needed. It is helpful to think of it as a temporary workspace. However, your working memory has limited storage and capacity, and is thus easily susceptible to overload. This is especially true when you feel anxious – will your adviser or partner notice you are having difficulty running all those numbers in your head?

Focused attention: You are always very busy at work. You never have enough time to finish what needs to be done and are always doing three things at once. You make mistakes and have to redo a lot of your work. What is going on? Different brain functions allow us to either focus our attention exclusively on one task or divide it between multiple tasks. Since human attention is limited, trying to divide it between too many tasks necessarily results in performance errors.

Emotional self-regulation: You are discussing a project with a new client. The situation is difficult for two reasons. First, it is an important deal for your career and you are anxious to close it to your advantage. Second, the client is quite condescending. The pressure to succeed and the need to refrain from getting angry make it hard for you to think straight. This is because emotion and cognition are tightly interconnected. Controlling and managing emotion (including stress and anger) is crucial for performing successfully in anything.

These examples illustrate a common point: A healthy brain with well-developed capabilities is important for all aspects of life. Ultimately, the human brain has evolved to help us operate in complex, changing environments by continually learning and adapting. Successfully doing so involves a variety of interdependent brain functions and abilities.

Cognition has to do with how a person understands and acts in the world, and cognitive skills are the brain-based processing capacities we need to carry out any task, from the simplest to the most complex. They have to do with the mechanisms of how we learn, remember, problem-solve, and pay attention. Any task can be broken down into a set of different cognitive skills or functions needed to complete that task successfully.

Emotions are complex states that involve both a physiological, or bodily, experience and a psychological, or cognitive, experience. They are closely related to motivation as they often precede our actions (e.g., if you are angry you may start arguing) or follow them (e.g., you may feel happy after helping someone). Feelings are part of the emotional experience: they are the way we consciously perceive and describe emotions.

Cognition and emotion are both critical parts of normal functioning. As neatly summarized by Dr. Robert Sylwester (whose interview can be found at the end of this chapter): "Emotion is the system that tells us how important something is. Attention focuses us on the important and away from the unimportant things. Cognition tells us what to do about it. Cognitive skills are whatever it takes to do those things."

In Table 1, you can browse through examples of different daily experiences and the brain functions and skills they involve. For more discussion of one crucial brain ability, attention, and how to enhance it, you can read the interview at the end of this chapter with Dr. Michael Posner, a pioneer in this area.

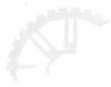

Daily experience	Brain Function	Skills involved
When you feel the cold of the snow, smell chocolate, recognize a picture, pat a cat, or taste a new dish.	Perception	Recognition and interpretation of sensory information.
When you block out distractions and immerse yourself in a good book (focused attention). When you answer the phone while following a program on TV (divided attention).	Attention	Ability to sustain concentration on a particular object, action, or thought. Ability to manage competing demands in our environment.
When you recall the phone number you just heard (STM). When you remember what you did that summer four years ago (LTM).	Memory	Short-term memory (STM) (limited storage). Long-term memory (LTM) (practically unlimited storage).
Whenever you move any parts of your body automatically (when you walk) or voluntarily (when you write).	Motor	Ability to mobilize our muscles and bodies. Ability to manipulate objects.
When you manage to hold a conversation during a loud party, write a paragraph for a report, or learn a new language.	Language and Auditory Processing	Skills allowing us to differentiate and comprehend sounds and generate verbal output.
When you recognize the logo of your favorite store or remember the face of a loved one. When you drive and manage the locations of both your car and the cars around you.	(Higher-order) Visual and Spatial Processing	Ability to process incoming visual information and visualize images and scenarios. Ability to process spatial relationships between objects.
When you realize that the method you were using to convince your child to listen to you may not be the best and decide to try the technique you read about recently instead (Flexibility). When you can feel the joy and imagine the thoughts of your coworker who just got a promotion (Theory of mind). When you keep in mind all the potential expenses involved in a trip while deciding where to go on your next vacation (Working memory).	Executive Functions	Abilities that enable goal-oriented behavior, such as the ability to plan, and execute a goal. These include: • Flexibility: the capacity for quickly switching to a different mental mode, revising plans, adapting. • Theory of mind: insight into other people's inner worlds, including their plans and their likes and dislikes. • Anticipation: prediction based on pattern recognition. • Problem-solving: defining the problem in the right way to then generate solutions and pick the right one.

Daily experience	Brain Function	Skills involved
When you realize that you are very angry and this is not going to help in the upcoming discussion with your partner, and decide to take a few deep breaths before entering the room (Emotional self-regulation). When you weigh the pros and cons of staying at your current position versus applying for a new job in a new city (Decision making). When you decide to refrain from eating that chocolate bar because this would be against your diet rules (Inhibition).	Executive Functions	• Decision making: the ability to make decisions based on problem-solving, on incomplete information, and on emotions (both ours and others'). • Working memory: the capacity to hold in mind and manipulate information in real time. • Emotional self-regulation: the ability to identify and manage one's own emotions. • Sequencing: the ability to break down complex actions into manageable units and prioritize them in the right order. • Inhibition: the ability to withstand distractions and internal urges.

TABLE 1. Main brain functions.

WHAT DO NEURONS DO?

These functions are ultimately produced by interacting cells in the brain. An average brain contains a staggering number of individual brain cells (known as "neurons;" see Figure 1) – approximately 100 billion of them. (Another category of cells, called glial cells, are even more numerous, and help neurons function normally.) Neurons have a specialized ability to manage bioelectrical information, and to communicate with each other by exchanging chemical information in the form of neurotransmitters (e.g. dopamine) through connections with other neurons, known as synapses. Each neuron can have up to 10,000 synapses with other neurons, for a total of many hundreds of trillions of neuronal connections in the brain as a whole.

All brain functioning is the result of neurons exchanging information, and the functions we depend on emerge from large groups of connected neurons working together as networks. For instance, moving your hand to turn the page is only possible because a network of neurons responsible for this command all start firing together in your frontal lobe when you decide to do so. In the same way, when you try to remember what you did last Monday morning, networks of neurons in the temporal and frontal lobes start firing and exchanging information.

Such networks of neurons are built following the principle that "cells that fire together, wire together" (Hebb's rule). In short, neurons that are frequently active at the same time tend to become associated and end up connecting with one another. This principle has major implications for brain fitness. First, the more a network of neurons is activated (i.e., the more often the neurons fire together), the stronger the connections become. If a network supporting a brain function is repeatedly stimulated through practice and training, it will become stronger, contributing to the optimization of that brain function. Second, by contrast, the less a network of neurons is activated the weaker the connections become, and weak connections end up dying. This accounts for the popular idea "use it or lose it" – brain functions that are not stimulated end up losing their efficiency since the neural networks supporting them weaken or dissipate.

These mechanisms, which result in an efficient allocation of limited neuronal resources, are why our genetic inheritances, while influencing how our brains and mental faculties develop during our lives, do not determine them completely. When it comes to your brain's structure and functioning, genes are far from the final word (more on that shortly).

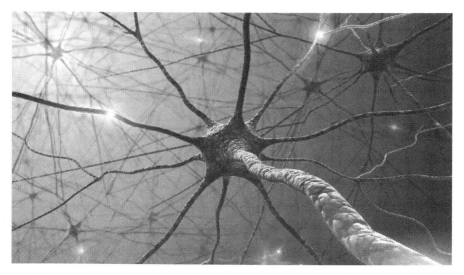

FIGURE 1. This is an illustration of a neuron. Your brain contains approximately 100 billion of them. Neurons communicate with each other through synapses.

HOW IS THE BRAIN STRUCTURED?

To summarize so far, our thoughts, feelings, and actions depend on a diverse collection of cognitive and emotional functions and skills, such as attention and working memory. These brain functions are themselves supported by networks of interconnected neurons that are "wired" together depending on how often those neurons fire at the same time. We are now ready to take a big picture look at the brain to see (at a simplified level) which networks and regions of networks support which functions.

The human brain consists of several main parts, including the brain stem, the cerebellum, the limbic system, and the neocortex. Structurally, the brain stem is at the bottom of the brain (in white in Fig. 2, mostly concealed), and the cerebellum rests somewhat behind it (the striped oval in Fig. 2). Moving up we encounter the limbic system on the inside, and the grey, curly cortex on the outside (the large, wrinkled, grey mass in Fig. 2). Almost all brain structures come in pairs, with one in the left hemisphere and one in the right hemisphere, and the two hemispheres constantly work together to manage mental functioning.

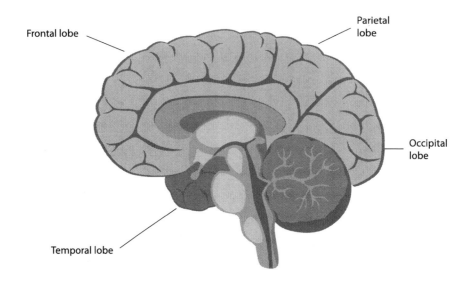

Frontal lobe

Parietal lobe

Occipital lobe

Temporal lobe

FIGURE 2. The cortex consists of two hemispheres, each divided into four lobes: frontal, parietal, occipital and temporal.

The brain stem relays information from the body to the rest of the brain, and is involved in the control of many basic functions (such as cardiovascular, respiratory, and pain functions). The cerebellum, among other things, plays a major role in motor control. The limbic system is composed of several structures (including the amygdala, the hippocampus, and the hypothalamus) that collaborate to process emotions, regulate memories, produce hormones, and manage sexual arousal and circadian rhythms. Specifically, the hippocampus plays a major role in memory, while the amygdala plays a major role in emotion. The neocortex ("new cortex") is the outer layer of each hemisphere and controls a variety of higher mental functions, such as perceptual processing, attention, and decision making. In each hemisphere, the neocortex and (most of) the limbic system can be divided into four distinct areas or lobes: the occipital, temporal, parietal, and frontal lobes.

Brain Function	Brain structures primarily involved
Perception	Vision: Occipital lobes and temporal lobes
	Hearing, smell, taste: Temporal lobes
	Touch: Parietal lobes
Attention	Parietal and frontal lobes
Memory	All of the neocortex and the hippocampi
Motor	Frontal lobes
Language and Auditory Processing	Temporal, parietal, and frontal lobes
Higher-order Visual and Spatial Processing	Visual processing: Mostly occipital lobes (with some help from the temporal and parietal lobes)
	Spatial processing: Parietal lobes
Executive Functions	Frontal lobes

TABLE 2. The main cortical functions and their supporting structures.

THE BRAIN THROUGHOUT LIFE

Our brains constantly change over the lifetime as we develop and age. As a consequence, the way various brain functions work also changes, sometimes for better and sometimes for worse.

The brain of a newborn is far from developed; it needs time to fully grow and establish connections on both large and small scales. Our brain's functions improve drastically throughout childhood and adolescence, following a generally predictable progression. It is only in our early 20's, or possibly even later, that we finally possess a fully-equipped brain, complete with a well-developed prefrontal cortex to help each of us succeed in leading an independent life as an adult.

Even after the brain is fully formed in young adulthood, researchers have found that functions that benefit from accumulated experience, such as vocabulary-related language skills, pattern recognition, and emotional self-regulation, tend to improve decade after decade. For example, Igor Grossmann and his colleagues asked individuals from three age groups (25–40, 41–59, and 60+) to read stories about intergroup and interpersonal conflicts and predict how these conflicts would unfold. Compared to young and middle-aged people, older people employed higher reasoning schemes that involved multiple perspectives, allowed for compromise, and recognized the limits of knowledge.

On the other hand, starting in our late 20's and early 30's, the research shows that speed of processing and working memory tend (on average) to slow down, reducing our capacity to process and deal with complex new information. This is a gradual process that often first becomes noticeable in our early 40's. For example, in a study published in 2012, Archana Singh-Manoux and her colleagues assessed the memory, comprehension and vocabulary skills of 7,000 men and women aged 45 to 70, three times over 10 years. They found that memory and comprehension abilities declined further at each decade.

This age-related slowing down happens in functions that underlie our capacity to learn quickly and adapt to new environments, such as problem-solving in novel situations, working memory, focused attention, inhibition, and flexibility. Of course, that is not to say that it renders any further learning and adapting impossible. Furthermore, individuals vary significantly in how and when they experience these decreases: some people experience a significant decline while others do not.

In short, old dogs can certainly learn – faster than young dogs in domains that benefit from accumulated experience, and slower in domains that change too rapidly for accumulated experience to accrue a significant benefit.

LIFELONG NEUROPLASTICITY

Most of what we have discussed in this chapter so far has been known for decades. What is new, and constitutes such a profound shift in our understanding of the human brain that society hasn't yet fully absorbed the implications, is scientific evidence from the past few decades that sheds light on the brain's potential for change and improvement throughout life.

How the brain can change at any age – for good, or for bad

Traditional scientific ideas cast the human brain as a fixed and essentially limited system that only degrades with age. This view saw the brain as a rigid machine in many ways, pretty much set after childhood. By contrast, we have now come to appreciate that the human brain is actually a highly dynamic and constantly reorganizing system, capable of being shaped and reshaped across the entire lifespan. It is believed that every experience alters the brain's organization at some level. The central concept in this new approach is neuroplasticity, the brain's lifelong capacity to change and rewire itself in response to the stimulation of learning and experience. This includes both the lifelong ability to create new neurons – neurogenesis – and to create new connections between neurons – synaptogenesis.

In a young brain, neuroplasticity, including neurogenesis and synaptogenesis, allows for fast learning, as well as for potentially faster repair. As we age, the rate of neuroplasticity declines, but does not come to a halt. As Dr. James Zull puts it: "We now know that every brain can change, at any age. There is really no upper limit on learning since the neurons seem to be capable of growing new connections whenever they are used repeatedly." (You can find Dr. Zull's interview at the end of this chapter.)

Lifelong neuroplasticity has major consequences for brain health and fitness. At a basic level, it means that our lifestyles and actions play a meaningful role in how our brains physically change throughout life. More specifically, neuroplasticity gives us the power to resist the effects of decline or disease by supporting our ability to accumulate knowledge and experiences, i.e., to learn. Learning helps to increase the so-called brain reserve (also known as cognitive reserve; more about it in Chapter 4) and strengthen the brain against age-related decline and potential dementia pathology by increasing the connections between neurons, increasing cellular metabolism, and increasing the production of nerve growth factor, a substance produced by the body to help maintain and repair neurons.

Furthermore, neuroplasticity not only enables us to prevent future cognitive decline but also provides a basis for a more optimistic outlook when it comes to our ability to address existing deficits, such as learning difficulties and recovery after traumatic brain injury or stroke. And finally, beyond preventing decline and overcoming deficits, neuroplasticity is at the core of the ability to actively improve our brains through brain training. By practicing a skill, one can repeatedly stimulate the same area of the brain, which strengthens existing neural connections and creates new ones. Over time, the brain can become more efficient, requiring less effort to do the same job.

Brain imaging provides examples of neuroplasticity

A key contributor to our growing understanding of large-scale neuroplasticity was the development of high-level brain imaging technologies. By allowing scientists to produce images of the brain that show its structure, as well as where activity spikes as it is engages in various cognitive activities, these neuroimaging methods have revolutionized neuroscience in the same way that the telescope revolutionized astronomy.

A little background here. There are two types of brain imaging: structural and functional. Structural imaging provides information about the shape and volume of the brain and its constituent regions, and includes computed axial tomography (CAT) and magnetic resonance imaging (MRI). Functional imaging, which includes functional magnetic resonance imaging (fMRI), positron emission tomography (PET), and Single Photon Emission Computerized Tomography (SPECT), shows patterns of brain activity, allowing researchers and clinicians to identify which regions see a spike in activity when an individual performs a specific task, as well as to examine patterns of regional brain activity in resting states. We can also study connectivity patterns between different brain regions; structural connectivity can be studied with a specialized form of MRI called Diffusion Tensor or Diffusion Kutrosis Imaging (DTI/DKI), while functional connectivity can be studied with fMRI.

Evidence of neuroplasticity gleaned from brain imaging has come mostly from the brains of individuals who became experts in a particular skill. Why? Because, as you might have guessed, changes associated with learning occur massively when we become expert in a specific function or domain.

For example, a fascinating 2006 study showed that London taxi drivers have a larger hippocampus than London bus drivers. This is explained by the fact that the hippocampus is important for forming and accessing complex memories, including the spatial memories necessary for efficient navigation. Taxi drivers have to navigate around London whereas bus drivers follow a limited set of routes. Thus, the hippocampus of a taxi driver is particularly stimulated and changes over time as a result.

Plasticity can also be observed in the brains of bilinguals. It looks like learning a second language is directly associated with structural changes in the brain: a region called the left inferior parietal cortex is larger in bilingual brains than in monolingual brains. Plastic changes have also been found to occur in musicians' brains (compared to non-musicians), with areas involved in playing music (motor regions, anterior superior parietal areas, and inferior temporal areas) showing increased volume.

These changes do not require a lifetime to occur; a few years can be enough. In a follow-up to the taxi drivers study published in 2011, the same researchers studied adults training to become licensed taxi drivers in London. The trainees' brain structures and memory performance were compared to those of non-taxi driver controls. The study lasted 4 years, the time it takes for taxi driver trainees to learn approximately 25,000 streets and their layout as well as 20,000 landmarks. At the end of the learning process all trainees took a series of exams that only about half passed. To start with, taxi driver trainees and non-taxi driver controls showed no differences in either brain structure or memory. Three to four years later, the size of the posterior hippocampus had increased in the brains of trainees who qualified as taxi drivers. These changes were not observed in trainees who failed to qualify, or in the non-taxi driver controls.

Other studies show that plastic changes in the brain can even be observed after just a few months. For instance, in 2006, researchers imaged the brains of German medical students three months before their medical exam, and again right after the exam, and then compared the brains of these students to the brains of students who were not studying for the exam at this time. The results: Medical students' brains showed changes in regions of the parietal cortex as well as in the posterior hippocampus. As you can probably guess, these regions are known to be involved in memory and learning.

Don't count on miracles

The large-scale changes observed in these studies were the result of serious effort over time, be it learning the streets of London or studying for a medical exam. It would be nice, of course, if we could all just take a pill to quickly and painlessly increase brain fitness: to suddenly become more attentive, never forget a name, and perform all the mental math we want. However, despite large investments, evidence that "smart" drugs actually work is scarce at the present. The recent extensive NIH meta-analysis (mentioned in the Introduction) found no evidence that any of the medications tracked (namely statins, antihypertensive medications, cholinesterase inhibitors, or estrogen) were successful at improving or maintaining cognitive functioning over time. Some drugs have produced positive effects for people who have neurological disorders such as Alzheimer's disease, Parkinson's disease, or Attention Deficit Disorder – when patients take these drugs, their symptoms are usually lessened. However, no solid scientific evidence has shown so far that these drugs are reliably beneficial or safe for people with normal functioning. Even in the supposed scenario that a smart drug that can "double brainpower" with no side effects is discovered, it would be misguided to believe that the drug alone would be enough. If things worked that way, why do steroid-taking athletes still have to pay attention to their physical exercise regimens?

What *is* supported by ample evidence is the brain's capacity to be flexible and be molded through experience. The question then becomes: "What activities or behaviors can provide the right kind of experience to help optimize my brain, from a structural and functional point of view?" The goal of the next chapters in this book is to help you answer that precise question.

CHAPTER HIGHLIGHTS

- We need to expand our vocabulary: "IQ" and "memory" do not encompass all of the brain's functions. The brain is composed of neuronal networks serving distinct functions, including various types of memory, but also language, emotional regulation, attention, planning, and many others. This is important because our life and productivity depend on the functionality of all these brain functions, not just one.

- The plasticity of the human brain refers to its lifelong capacity to change and reorganize itself in response to the stimulation of learning and experience. Education, lifestyle, and decisions under our control matter as much as our genetic inheritance in the trajectory of our mental capacity over time.

INTERVIEWS

- Dr. Robert Sylwester – Cognition and brain development.

- Dr. James Zull – What is learning?

- Dr. Michael Posner – What is attention and how to train it.

Interview with Dr. Robert Sylwester – Cognition and brain development.

BACKGROUND:

Dr. Robert Sylwester is an educator of educators. He has received multiple awards during his long career as a master communicator of the implications of brain science research for education and learning. He is the author of several books and many journal articles, and a member of SharpBrains' Scientific Advisory Board. His most recent books are *The*

Adolescent Brain: Reaching for Autonomy (2007) and *A Child's Brain: The Need for Nurture* (2010). He is an Emeritus Professor of Education at the University of Oregon.

HIGHLIGHTS:

- ⮑ Significant human brain development happens after birth: Humans are born with an immature brain that develops mass and capabilities during 20 year after birth.

- ⮑ Our brains are plastic: Every experience alters the brain's organization at some level.

LEARNING AND COGNITION

Let us start by defining some words such as learning, education, brain development and cognition.

Most organisms begin life with all of the processing systems and information that they need to survive. Humans are a notable exception in that an adult-size brain is significantly larger than a mother's birth canal. So, we are born with an immature one pound brain that develops additional mass and capabilities during its twenty year post-birth developmental trajectory. Parenting, mentoring, teaching, and mass media are examples of the cultural systems that humans have developed to help young people master the knowledge and skills they need to survive and thrive in complex environments. Learning is one of the main activities we do, even if many times we are not aware of it.

Education, like the culture it subsumes, is a conservative phenomenon. Science and technology move rapidly, education does not. So if schools often resemble the schools of fifty years ago, that should not be surprising. Parents remember their school experiences, and since they survived them, they are typically leery about educators "experimenting" with their children. Which explains why, in general, schools have not incorporated many of the lessons from neuroscience and cognitive psychology.

Childhood brain development is focused on systems that allow children to recognize and remember the dynamics of environmental challenges – challenges that protective adults will solve for them. Adolescent brain development is more focused on frontal lobe development, the systems that allow us to respond appropriately and autonomously to the challenges we confront.

Every remembered experience will alter our brain's organization at some level. Our brain's processing networks continually change throughout our life – this process is called brain plasticity. For example, my brain has adapted to my switch from using a typewriter to using a computer. So, it would now be difficult for me to relearn how to write on a typewriter.

Emotion is the system that tells us how important something is. Attention focuses us on the important and away from the unimportant things. Cognition tells us what to do about it. Cognitive skills are whatever it takes to do those things.

ROLE OF NATURE VS. NURTURE IN BRAIN DEVELOPMENT

What are the respective roles of genes and our environment in brain development?

Genetic and environmental factors both contribute to brain maturation. Genetics probably play a stronger role in the early years, and the environment plays a stronger role in later years. Still development can be affected by the mother's use of drugs during a pregnancy (this is an environmental factor). Some adult illnesses, such as Huntington's Disease, are genetically triggered.

We typically think of environmental factors as things that happen to us, over which we have little control. Can our own decisions have an effect on our own brain development? For example, what if I choose a career in investment banking vs. one in journalism?

When we make our career decisions in life, most of us make a combination of good and bad decisions which have an influence on our brain maturation and development. My father was very unusual in his career trajectory in that he worked at one place throughout his entire adult life, and died three months after he retired at ninety-one years old. I have always thought that it is a good idea to make a change every ten years or so and do something different – either within the same organization or to move to another one. It is just as good for organizations to have some staff turnover as it is for staff to move to new challenges. The time to leave one position for another is while you and your employer are still happy with what you are doing.

In 2007 you published a book titled The Adolescent Brain. What advice would you give to parents and educators of adolescents?

Biological phenomena always operate within ranges. For example, leaves fall from trees in the autumn, but not all at once. Developmental changes similarly do not all occur at the same time and at the same rate in every child and adolescent brain. And just as it is possible for wind or temperature to alter the time when a leaf might fall, unexpected events can alter the time when an adolescent has to confront and respond to given environmental challenges. The important thing for adults to do is to carefully observe an adolescent's interests and abilities, and insert challenges that move maturation forward at a reasonable level. If you push too fast, you end up with a stressed out adolescent. If you do not challenge sufficiently, you end up with a bored adolescent. No magic formula exists for getting this just right. This means, for example, that we celebrate the skills of artists and athletes who function beyond typical human capacity, and we create judicial sanctions for those whose behavior does not reach culturally acceptable levels. Most human behavior is personally chosen and executed within wide ranges. We can easily observe this wide range in such phenomena as political discourse and religious belief or practice. Adolescents strive towards autonomous adulthood as they gradually discover their interests and capabilities, and what is biologically possible and culturally appropriate. They adapt their life to wherever they're most comfortable within the marvelous sets of possible and appropriate ranges that exist.

Adolescents take risks, no doubt about that. If you want to eventually function within any range, you have to locate its outer positive and negative limits. Speed limits and other regulations provide direction, but adolescents (and adults) still tend to move towards the limits – and maybe just a smidge beyond. Bad things can then occur. Parents and educators need to pay attention to observe where adolescents' interests and abilities lie and actively engage them with experiences that will enable them to move forward.

There is a constant debate in education on whether we should focus efforts on nurturing all of the so-called "multiple intelligences," as defined by Howard Gardner, or focus on our strengths. What is your opinion?

Let me know when you have figured out the correct answer to this conundrum and I will contact the folks in Stockholm who give out the Nobel Prizes.

BRAIN RESOURCES

What are the most exciting areas of brain research, and what are some resources such as websites or books for educators to learn about the brain to refine their teaching?

The cognitive neurosciences are currently so dynamic that it seems like an exciting new development occurs every day, and many of these new developments are reported in the mass media. I used to write a monthly non-technical column on educationally significant developments in the cognitive neurosciences for the Internet journal Brain Connection. www.Sharpbrains.com is another great resource.

What is one recent finding or reflection, from your own work or others', that you'd like more people of all ages to know about as they try to maintain/enhance their own brain fitness?

Perhaps the most intriguing recent development in my own life involves mystery novels. It dawned on me that a good mystery novel has a complex plot and characters. It thus forces us to hold all of this in mind as we read the novel and use our prefrontal cortex to predict the ending — plot twists and turns, character development, location, etc. I thus decided to read a series of mystery novels to see how it would affect my mind and memory. Reading a related series of books in sequence gets one deeper into the characters and the procedures they use to solve the mystery.

I wanted to locate an exceptionally well-done series and then basically read it straight through. Fortunately, the Stieg Larsson's Millenium trilogy had just been published in English, so I read it while I was bedridden for three weeks. It was such an intellectually stimulating experience that I sought out other highly rated series that would actively stimulate my thinking capabilities.

My next series was the superb 11 book Inspector Kurt Wallender series by Henning Mankell, which also takes place in Sweden. I thus read two excellent sets of novels and learned a lot about Sweden and the human condition in the process. Another fine mystery series by James Lee Burke involves a New Orleans area police officer, Dave Robicheaux. Great descriptive writing. My parents grew up in Minnesota, so John Sandford's Virgil Flowers series was another fascinating set with personal interest. I've just begun the Norwegian 10 book Inspector Sejer series by Karin Fossum, so it's obvious that I've discovered something that has worked well to enhance my mind and memory beyond the professional reading and writing that I continue to do.

My advice if you're not a regular mystery buff: use the Internet to locate a highly respected author who gets beyond potboiler novels into complex characters and plots. Get and read the whole series, but only buy the first two of the novels initially to see if they stimulate your thought. Most series books will now be inexpensively available in used book stores, or free in your local library. Get a map of the locations where the novel is located, and Google the town — so that you're comfortable with the novel's background. I suspect that you'll discover as I did, that a series of mystery novels can be a relaxing and intellectually stimulating experience. You might begin with one of the excellent series I identified above.

Interview with Dr. James Zull – What is learning?

BACKGROUND:

Dr. James Zull is a Professor of biology and biochemistry at Case Western University. Dr. Zull is also the Director of the University Center for Innovation in Teaching and Education (UCITE) at Case Western. Dr. Zull loves to learn, teach, and build connections. He has spent years building bridges between neurobiology and pedagogy. His book, *The Art of Changing the Brain: Enriching the Practice of Teaching by Exploring the Biology of Learning*, shows how neurobiological research can inform and refine some of the best ideas in educational theory. In the book, Dr. Zull adds a biological perspective to David Kolb's Learning Cycle framework from his book, *Experiential Learning: Experience as the Source of Learning and Development*. Whereas Kolb reviews human learning, Dr. Zull is focused on how apes go through the same stages when they learn a new activity, activating exactly the same brain areas that we do.

HIGHLIGHTS:

- Every brain can change, at any age, so learning is critical at all ages, not only in the school environment.

- Children need to flex their "learning muscle" – to learn how to learn.

- Schools should focus more on how all kids could learn more.

THE VIRTUOUS LEARNING CYCLE

What is learning? Can apes really learn the same way that humans do?

Learning is physical. Learning means the modification, growth, and pruning of our neuronal networks, through experience. And, yes, we have seen that apes go through the same Learning Cycle that we do, activating the same or similar brain areas.

How does learning happen?

There are 4 stages in the "Learning Cycle:"
Stage One: We have a concrete experience.
Stage Two: We develop reflective observations and connections.
Stage Three: We generate abstract hypotheses
Stage Four: Then we actively test those hypotheses.

In the fourth stage, we have a new concrete experience, and a new Learning Cycle ensues. In other words, we get information (activating the sensory cortex), make meaning of that information (in the back integrative cortex), create new ideas from these meanings (in the front integrative cortex), and act on those ideas (using the motor cortex). From this, I propose that there are four pillars of learning: gathering, analyzing, creating, and acting. This is how we learn.

Learning in this way requires effort and getting out of our comfort zones. A key condition for learning is self-driven motivation, a sense of ownership. To feel in control, to feel that one is making progress, is necessary for this Learning Cycle to self-perpetuate. Antonio Damasio made a strong point about the role of emotions in his engaging book *Descartes' Error*.

HOW TO IMPROVE LEARNING ABILITIES

Can we, as learners, motivate ourselves? How can we become better learners?

Great question, because in fact that is a uniquely human ability. We know that the brain's frontal lobes, which are proportionally much larger in humans than in any other mammals, are key for emotional self-regulation. We can be proactive and identify the areas that motivate us, and build on those. In other words, the "art of the learner" may be the art of finding connections between the new information or challenges and what we already know and care about.

If I had to select one mental muscle that students should really exercise and grow during their school years, I would say they need to build their "learning muscle" – to learn how to learn. That might be even more valuable than learning what we stress in the curriculum, i.e., rote memory and the specific subjects we teach.

Do you think this is happening today in schools?

I do not think so. First, of all, too many people still believe that education means the process by which students passively absorb information. Even if many educators would like to ensure a more participatory and active approach, we still use the structures and priorities of another era. For example, we still pay too much attention to categorizing some kids as intelligent and some as not so intelligent, instead of focusing on how all kids could learn more.

Second, learning and changing are not that easy. Both require effort, and also, by definition, getting out of our comfort zones. We need to try new things, and to fail. The active testing phase is a critical one.

Sometimes our hypothesis will be right, and sometimes it will be wrong. The fear of failing, the fear of looking not smart, is a key obstacle to learning that I see too often, especially with people who want to protect perceived reputations to such an extent that they do not let themselves try new learning cycles.

Given what you just said, how do you help your students become better learners?

Despite the fact that every brain is different, let me simplify and say that I usually observe two types of students each with different obstacles to learning and benefiting from different strategies.

1. Introverted Students: Students who have a tendency toward introversion can be very good at the reflection and abstract hypothesis phases, but not so good at the active testing one. In order to change that, I help create small groups where they feel safe and can take risks such as sharing their thoughts aloud and asking questions.

2. Extroverted Students: More extroverted students can be very good at having constant concrete experiences and active testing, but may benefit from increased reflection and abstract hypothesis development. Having them do things like writing papers and predicting the outcome of certain experiments or even current political affairs, helps.

What other tips would you offer to teachers and parents to help children learn?

Always try to provoke an active reaction. This will ensure that the student is engaged and sees the connection between the new information and what he or she already knows. You can do this by asking questions such as "What does this make you think of? Is there some part of this new material that rings a bell for you?"

To ensure a safe learning environment, you have to make sure to accept all answers, and build on them. We should view students as plants and flowers that need careful cultivation: grow some areas, help reduce others.

Please give us an example.

An example I use in my books is that middle school students often have a hard time learning about Martin Luther and the Reformation because they confuse him with Martin Luther King Jr. We can choose to become frustrated about that. Or we can exploit this saying something like, "Yes! Martin Luther King was a lot like Martin Luther. In fact, why do you think Martin Luther King's parents named him that? Why do you think they did not name him Sam King?"

LEARNING AND THE ADULT BRAIN

What would you suggest for adults who want to become better learners?

Learning is critical at all ages, not only in the school environment. We have brains precisely in order to be able to learn, to adapt to new environments. This is essential throughout life, not just when we are in school.

We now know that every brain can change, at any age. There is really no upper limit on learning since the neurons seem to be capable of growing new connections whenever they are used repeatedly. I think all of us need to develop the capacity to motivate ourselves. One way to do that is to search for meaningful contact points and bridges, between what we want to learn and what we already know. When we do so, we cultivate our neuronal networks. We become our own gardeners.

Interview with Dr. Michael I. Posner –
What is attention and how to train it

BACKGROUND:

Michael I. Posner is a prominent scientist in the field of cognitive neuroscience. He is currently an Emeritus Professor of Neuroscience at the University of Oregon (Department of Psychology, Institute of Cognitive and Decision Sciences). In August 2008, the International Union of Psychological Science made him the first recipient of the Dogan Prize in recognition of a contribution that represents a major advance in psychology.

HIGHLIGHTS:

- There is not one single "attention," but three separate functions of attention: alerting, orienting, and executive attention.

- A 5-day intervention aimed at training executive attention in children between 4 and 7 years of age showed that executive attention was trainable.

Dr. Posner, many thanks for your time today. I really enjoyed the James Arthur Lecture monograph on Evolution and Development of Self-regulation that you delivered last year. Could you provide a Summary of the research you presented?

I would emphasize that we human beings can regulate our thoughts, emotions, and actions to a greater degree than other primates. For example, we can choose to pass up an immediate reward for a larger, delayed reward. We can plan ahead, resist distractions, be goal-oriented. These human characteristics appear to depend upon what we often call "self-regulation." What is exciting these days is that progress in neuroimaging and in genetics makes it possible to think about self-regulation in terms of specific brain-based networks.

Can you explain what self-regulation is?

All parents have seen this in their kids. Parents can see the remarkable transformation as their children develop the ability to regulate emotions and to persist with goals in the face of distractions. That ability is usually labeled "self-regulation."

The other main area of your research is attention. Can you explain the brain basis for what we usually call "attention"?

I have been interested in how the attention system develops in infancy and early childhood. One of our major findings, thanks to neuroimaging, is that there is not one single "attention," but three separate functions of attention with three separate underlying brain networks: alerting, orienting, and executive attention.

1. Alerting: helps us maintain an alert state.
2. Orienting focuses our senses on the information we want. For example, you are now listening to my voice.

3. Executive Attention: regulates a variety of networks, such as emotional responses and sensory information. This is critical for most other skills, and clearly correlated with academic performance. It is distributed in frontal lobes and the cingulate gyrus. The development of executive attention can be easily observed both by questionnaire and cognitive tasks after about age 3-4, when parents can identify the ability of their children to regulate their emotions and control their behavior in accord with social demands.

"Executive attention" sounds similar to executive functions.

Executive functions are goal-oriented. Executive attention is just the ability to manage attention towards those goals, towards planning. Both are clearly correlated. Executive attention is important for decision-making (how to accomplish an external goal) and with working memory (the temporary storage of information). For example, given that you said earlier that you liked my monograph, I have been thinking of the subheadings and sections there as I provide you my answers, using my working memory capacity.

You said that the three functions of attention are supported by separate neural networks.

Neuroimaging allows us to identify sets of distributed areas that operate together. Different techniques allow us to see different things. For example, fMRI lets us see the activation of areas of grey matter. A more recent technique, diffusion tensor, is focused instead on the white matter. It detects connectivity among neurons, it helps us see a map of networks.

How many networks have been identified so far?

So far, a number of networks have been identified. For an illustration, you can see the wonderful interactive Brain Map by the University of Texas, San Antonio. Let me add another fascinating area of research. There is a type of neuron, named the Von Economo neuron, which is found only in the anterior cingulate and a related area of the anterior insula, very common in humans, less in other primates, and completely absent in most non-primates. These neurons have long axons, connecting to the anterior cingulate and anterior insula, which we think is part of the reason why we have Executive Attention. Diffusion tensor allows us to identify this white matter, these connections across separate brain structures, in the live brain. From a practical point of view, we can think that neural networks like this are what enable specific human traits such as effortful control.

What is effortful control?

It is a higher-order temperament factor consisting of attention, focus shifting, and inhibitory control – both for children and adults. A common example is how often you may make plans that you do not follow through with. A test often used to measure executive attention is the Stroop Test.

Effortful control has been shown to correlate with the scores on executive attention at several ages during childhood, and imaging studies have linked it to brain areas involved in self-regulation. Good parenting has been shown to build good effortful control, so there are clear implications from this research.

Tell us now about your recent research on attention training.

Several training programs have been successful in improving attention in normal adults and in patients suffering from different pathologies. With normal adults, training with video games produced better performance on a range of visual attention tasks. Training has also led to specific improvements in executive attention in patients with specific brain injury. Working-memory training can improve attention with ADHD children.

In one study we developed and tested a 5-day training intervention using computerized exercises. We tested the effect of training during the period of major development of executive attention, which takes place between 4 and 7 years of age. We found that executive attention was trainable, and also a significantly greater improvement in intelligence in the trained group compared to the control children. This finding suggested that training effects had generalized to a measure of cognitive processing that is far removed from the training exercises.

A collaborator of our lab, Dr. Yiyuan Tang, studied the impact of mindfulness meditation with undergraduates to improve executive attention, finding significant improvements as well. We hope that training methods like this will be further evaluated, along with other methods, both as possible means of improving attention prior to school and for children and adults with specific needs.

Can you explain the potential implications of this emerging research on education and health?

It is clear that executive attention and effortful control are critical for success in school. Will they one day be trained in pre-schools? It sounds reasonable to believe so, to make sure all kids are ready to learn. Of course, additional studies are needed to determine exactly how and when attention training can best be accomplished and its lasting importance.

In terms of health, many deficits and clinical problems have a component of serious deficits in executive attention network. For example, when we talk about attention deficits, we can expect that in the future there will be remediation methods, such as working memory training, to help alleviate those deficits.

Let me add that we have found no ceiling for abilities such as attention, including among adults. The more training, even with normal people, the higher the results.

Let me ask your take on that eternal question, the roles of nature and nurture.

There is a growing number of studies that show the importance of interaction between our genes and each of our environments. Epigenetics is going to help us understand that question better, but let me share a very interesting piece of research from my lab where we found an unusual interaction between genetics and parenting.

Good parenting, as measured by different research-based scales, has been shown to build good effortful control which, as we saw earlier, is so important. Now, what we found is that some specific genes reduced, even eliminated, the influence of the quality of parenting. In other words, some children's development really depends on how their parents bring them up, whereas others do not – or do to a much smaller extent.

Too bad that we do not have time now to explore all the potential ethical implications from emerging research like that... Let me ask a few final questions. First, given that we have been talking both about formal training programs (computer-based, meditation) and also informal ones (parenting), do we know how formal and informal learning interact? What type can be most effective when, and for whom?

Great question. We don't know at this point. A research institute in Seattle, funded by the National Science Foundation, is trying to address that question. One practical issue they address is the influence of bilingual education on cognition.

What is one recent finding or reflection, from your own work or others', that you'd like more people of all ages to know about as they try to maintain/enhance their own brain fitness?

Recently, we uncovered an important mechanism by which a month of mindfulness meditation (about 11 hours of practice, 0.5 per day, 5 days a week) improves attention and self-regulation (Tang et al 2010; 2012). This mechanism is a change in the white matter that conducts signals into and out of the anterior cingulate gyrus. The anterior cingulate is an important part of the system by which we can voluntarily regulate behavior. After two weeks of meditation the improvements seemed to involve the number of fibers conducting information. This improvement was related to more positive and less negative mood self-reports. After 4 weeks of meditation improvement in white matter involved changes in the myelin that provides insulation to the fibers and thus further increases the efficiency of the network involved in self-regulation.

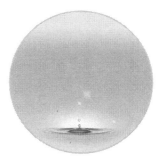

CHAPTER 2

BE A COACH, NOT A PATIENT

Brain fitness as a commonplace aspiration and culture is a recent development. The underlying scientific research is still fragmented and rapidly evolving. And while interest in emerging findings is high, they often fail to be channeled into accurate knowledge and actionable insights. Taking full advantage of the latest advances to positively impact your brain's health and fitness requires being ahead of the curve in sorting, understanding, and applying the newest scientific insights. This chapter will help you to navigate the growing scientific evidence and to apply these findings to your life.

THE FUTURE IS (ALMOST) HERE

There are several profound trends that one needs to understand in order to be ready for the future and to benefit from emerging brain research and tools, rather than be mystified or confused by them.

A focus on brain fitness naturally develops in step with an interest in assessment – targeted improvement requires the ability to compare functioning over time to measure change and set goals. As a result, we expect that better and more widely available assessments of cognitive function will soon serve as objective baselines to measure the impact of cognitive training interventions. There will also likely be better diagnostic tests to identify early symptoms of dementia. Reliable diagnostic assessments of cognitive abilities will help move this field forward in the same way that being able to jump on a scale to measure body weight is helpful in telling you if your physical fitness and diet program is working.

We can expect this increasing prevalence of brain fitness concepts and technologies to affect corresponding change in the way we deal with our brains in a healthcare context. Thus, we expect that psychologists and physicians will eventually help patients navigate the overwhelming assortment of available methodologies and interpret the results of cognitive assessments; health professionals will counsel their patients on tips for brain health in the same way they discuss various cardiac risk factors and how they can be addressed.

At the same time, employers and insurance companies are starting to introduce incentives for members to encourage optimization of brain health and performance. Many insurance plans today include rewards for members who, for example, voluntarily take health-related questionnaires that enable them to identify steps necessary to improve health; brain-related lifestyle factors will likely increasingly become a component of these interventions.

Attention to brain fitness is already increasing in locations ranging from retirement communities to gyms. As computer-savvy adults look for ways to stay mentally fit, brain fitness is becoming part of their vocabulary and concern. Physical and mental exercise traditionally take place in very different settings: the former in gyms and fitness clubs, the latter in school, or at work or home. In the coming years, we expect the boundaries between them to become more permeable, with the popularization of things like exercise bikes with built-in brain games and brain fitness podcasts that allow you to train working memory as you jog.

We feel confident these changes will happen because we can already see many such initiatives beginning to taking shape today. However, it always takes time for the newest scientific findings to make their full societal – including cultural and commercial – impact felt, and brain fitness is no exception. It may take at least a decade for brain fitness to attain the recognition, integration, and professional infrastructure that physical fitness enjoys today. Which is why we believe that, in the meantime, you will be best served by being able to coach yourself on how to optimize your brain health and performance.

DON'T OUTSOURCE YOUR BRAIN

High-quality scientific evidence of the kind that informs this book is a great starting point to guide learning and decision-making. But access to research results is not enough on its own. Applying those discoveries into smart decisions and valuable changes in your own life can be done much more effectively when you start with a basic framework with which to approach any particular piece of scientific evidence or personal decision. Here are a few pointers to help guide decisions in a meaningful way.

What are my priorities?

When the media covers brain health, the angle taken is often restricted to preventing the cognitive decline and Alzheimer's disease which may happen X number of years from now. Ignored are other important concerns such as improving functioning in all areas of life, years – if not decades – before the specter of AD appears on the horizon.

In practice, not everybody is interested in brain optimization for the same reasons. This is well illustrated by the results of a survey we performed. In 2010, SharpBrains eNewsletter subscribers (a self-selected assemblage of decision-makers and early adopters in the brain fitness field) were sent an online survey: 1,910 people responded to the detailed questionnaire. When asked about the brain functions they thought were the most important for thriving personally and professionally in the 21st century, their top three choices were: 1) the ability to manage stressful situations, 2) the concentration power to avoid distractions, and 3) being able to recognize and manage one's emotions (see Figure 3 below for their complete ranking of 10 brain functions). In other words, the priorities of the respondents seemed to focus around career and personal life at the *present* time; remembering faces and names, a common priority for someone worried about Alzheimer's disease, came in the last position.

With brain health and fitness goals varying widely between individuals, and over the lifespan within the same person, a crucial aspect of approaching scientific findings and effectively managing and making informed decisions about your brain fitness is taking into consideration what you, personally, want and need. Taking charge of you brain fitness begins with determining what your priorities are at the current time (more on this in Chapter 9).

How important do you believe the following brain functions are for thriving personally and professionally in the 21st Century?

Ranked from very important to less:

1. Ability to manage stressful situations
2. Concentration power to avoid distractions
3. Being able to recognize and manage one's emotions
4. Processing new information quickly
5. Defining and pursuing personally meaningful goals
6. Being able to monitor and manage one's thought processes
7. Ability to deal with new, uncertain situations
8. Planning ahead and solving problems in systematic ways
9. Ability to multi-task
10. Remembering faces and names

Figure 3. Partial results from 2010 SharpBrains Market Survey.

Is this relevant to me?

Another key aspect of informed brain health decision-making is getting accustomed to critically assessing new findings in order to stick with research of high quality and relevance. An important step in this process of deciding whether a specific piece of scientific evidence is of interest is to note in what population it was obtained. For instance, headlines regularly claim that a new medicine may help fight Alzheimer's disease. The inevitable result is that people build expectations and look for the new drug in stores in the near future without understanding that the actual findings are often not as relevant or significant as the headlines imply.

In February 2012, the news hit that a drug usually used to treat skin cancer had been shown to reverse the course of Alzheimer's disease in mice: within 72 hours after taking the drug, the mice showed dramatic improvements in memory and more than 50% of the amyloid protein accumulation in the brain (a hallmark of Alzheimer's disease) had disappeared. That is a quite dramatic result. But mice are not humans, and the mouse model of Alzheimer's disease is different from the actual disease in humans. What works in mice may fail to be effective in humans – just as dozens of promising theories and approaches have so failed in the past. So it is crucial to keep such results in perspective, and to prioritize high quality studies with humans.

Be aware of cognitive biases

Finally, good decision-making (in all matters) requires an awareness of the human tendency to rely on various cognitive biases when making decisions. Our brains, as you may remember from the previous chapter, evolved to help us learn and adapt – not to be objectively accurate. One consequence of the peculiarities of our mental processing systems is the persistence of reliable tendencies toward specific judgment errors, known as cognitive biases.

Here are three common biases:

The Exposure effect: This is the tendency to like things merely because they are familiar. For instance, having heard for decades that crossword puzzles or blueberries are the most important things to promote brain health may make them seem more convincing than they are. It can perhaps be explained by the fact that it takes less work for our brains to process things that are familiar.

Confirmation bias: This is the tendency to favor information that confirms one's preconceptions, beliefs, or hypotheses. For instance, having always believed that videogames are responsible for violent behaviors may lead a person to generally only notice, and therefore remember, news reports suggesting that videogames are bad for the brain. A more subtle example that we have witnessed often: A person reads a book (such as the one you hold in your hands) not to figure out what else he or she could be doing but simply to find reinforcement for whatever it is that person already believes and does, while ignoring the rest.

Recency bias: This is the tendency to overvalue and remember more vividly information that was encountered more recently. For instance, having read a news story yesterday may lead you to lend it more credence than the one you read last week – even if it was actually of worse quality. Imagine the combined impact of this natural bias with the barrage of daily news about brain health.

As you can imagine, it becomes that much harder to understand and navigate new information when people tend to favor information that is familiar, recent, and in accordance with prior beliefs. Since these biases can be present in people listening and reading as well as the people providing the information (e.g., a journalist or an "expert") the situation becomes even more muddied, especially in an area undergoing rapid change.

Knowing that these tendencies exist and understanding the way that they bias decisions is a step towards being able to counter their effects. Resources such as this book, and the framework we will present in Chapter 9, can be valuable for forcing us to rethink our assumptions and conclusions. The scientific process, when properly led and interpreted, is one of the most powerful tools at our disposal to make good decisions in any field – and especially in one as complex as brain health.

THE VALUE OF THE SCIENTIFIC PROCESS

In February 2012, a study published in the journal Therapeutic Advances in Psychopharmacology triggered a small wave of media reports with titles such as "How Sniffing Rosemary Could Boost Your Brain Power" or "Rosemary Brain Benefit: Study Shows Link Between

Herb Chemical And Brainpower". The study showed that after smelling rosemary, traces of a compound in the herb's oil (1,8-cineole) could be found in the blood of the study's participants. The more 1,8-cineole in the bloodstream of the person, the better the person's performance was on speed and accuracy tests.

We wouldn't be surprised if new rosemary herbal supplements became available in your local supermarket claiming to boost brain power. But numerous questions should come to mind when reading these headlines. How many people were involved? How big was the effect? How does it compare to previous studies, and were these results replicated by others?

This is just an example, but it illustrates an important point. Things have changed from the days when science was kept in the laboratories and new findings could take years to disseminate to the general public. Today, scientists, reporters, and companies that may have financed or stand to benefit from the findings all too frequently find themselves under more pressure to produce an exciting or provocative headline than to educate. And brain optimization seems to be very popular these days. What should one think about such raw findings? About how to pick and choose what information is most relevant or trustworthy? How to integrate new and old knowledge, and how to navigate options?

Observational and randomized controlled studies

When approaching new findings with a critical eye, a crucial element to evaluate is the design of the study behind the headline. The main difference of interest here is between observational studies and randomized controlled trials.

In observational studies, the researchers only observe associations (or correlations) between different factors and the behavior or disease they are interested in. This would be a study, for instance, looking at whether obesity is associated with cognitive deficits. Such a study could potentially show that there is a relation between obesity and lower performance in planning, reasoning and problem solving abilities. However, this does not imply a *causal* relationship between the two. Other factors, such as socio-economic factors, may be responsible for the observed association. Also the direction of the association is not clear: is it being obese that triggers cognitive deficits or does having such cognitive deficits increase one's likelihood of becoming obese? Many news stories that include the word "link" in the headline suffer from this problem and, while potentially interesting to read, can safely be ignored when we are making practical decisions.

By contrast, in a randomized controlled trial (RCT), each participant is randomly assigned to either a test group (where participants receive the intervention in question) or a control/placebo group (where they don't). This allows us to clearly evaluate the effect of the treatment or intervention in the test group by comparing it with the control/placebo group. For instance, a RCT could be conducted to measure the direct impact observed between meditation practice and better cognitive performance. Such a RCT could compare a group of participants using a particular meditation technique for 8 weeks to a (control) group of participants looking at educational videos for the same amount of time. If, after the training, the participants in the training group show better cognitive performance than the participants in the control group, then it is likely that the training (and not other factors) caused the increase in performance.

In sum, RCTs provide the most compelling evidence that a treatment or intervention indeed causes the expected effect on human health or behavior. There are of course many other nuances, such as the scientific quality of the journal in which the study was published, how durable the benefits were and which subgroup seemed to benefit the most, whether there was a disclosed or potential conflict of interest...but, at the very least, high-quality, randomized controlled trials offer a great place to begin making sense of the science and how to apply it.

Furthermore, even taking this into account, it is important to stay alert and to count on a solid previous understanding to contextualize new reported "findings."

The media challenge: BBC versus NIH studies

In April 2010, hundreds of media articles were published with titles like "Brain Training Doesn't Work" based on the "Brain Test Britain" experiment sponsored by the BBC. The study essentially showed that putting together a variety of non-validated "brain games" online and asking people under 60 (data from those over 60 was collected but surprisingly excluded from the analysis) who happen to show up to play around for a grand total of 3–4 hours over 6 weeks (10 minutes, three times a week, for six weeks) did not result in meaningful improvements in cognitive functioning. On this basis, the international headline became "Brain Training Doesn't Work."

The study was conducted through a BBC show's web site and involved 11,430 individuals. There were two experimental "brain training" groups. One completed tasks including simple arithmetic, finding missing pieces, matching symbols to a target, ordering rotating numbers, and memorizing items. The other group was trained on reasoning tasks (such as identifying relative weights of objects, selecting the "odd" item, thinking through the effects of one action, and planning tasks). The control group spent time answering questions about facts and organizing them chronologically based on any available online resource. Results indicated that among all the neuropsychological tests used before and after the training to assess cognitive abilities, the two experimental groups performed better than the control group on only one: a test of grammatical reasoning. There were no differences between either experimental groups and the control group on the other tests. In sum, the experimental groups improved on the trained tasks but this benefit did not transfer to non-trained tasks.

This study was criticized by a good number of scientists for obvious flaws in both methodology and interpretation – but that didn't make the news. First, the study occurred at home, so there was no control over what the participants were doing while training (maybe watching TV), a condition which usually produces "noisy" data. Second, there was a substantial, unexplained dropout rate: of 52,617 participants who registered, approximately only 20% completed full participation in the study. This brings into question the generalizability of the results: perhaps the people who dropped out were people who could have benefited from the training? Then, there is the fact that the training protocol was designed to be very light (3h-4h over six weeks) compared to what has been shown in other studies to produce measurable benefits (at least 10-15 hours per targeted cognitive domain). Even more surprisingly, only younger participants were included in the final analysis. The fatal flaw in terms of interpretation came from drawing a general conclusion from a single negative result. It amounted to manufacturing a car that didn't work, and then concluding that cars in general do not work.

As a consequence, one cannot conclude from the BBC study that brain training does not work (it can work when basic "conditions for transfer" are met, as we'll discuss in Chapter 8). And we can learn the larger lesson that it is unrealistic to expect the popular media to serve as a dependable source of quality education – for better or worse, that is simply not its primary role.

Now consider the systematic meta-analytic study on the prevention of cognitive decline and Alzheimer's disease commissioned by the National Institute of Health (NIH), which was published after the BBC study. The authors analyzed the results of 25 reviews of studies and 250 specific studies to understand which factors are associated with the reduction of risks of Alzheimer's disease and cognitive decline in older adults. The criteria to include a study in the analysis were very strict and only high-quality studies (mostly RCTs) were used, and of those, only studies that measured benefits (or lack thereof) over time. This is crucial since it makes the results of the analysis very conservative: if a positive result is found then it is probably real – at least more real than other interventions which didn't make the cut. The NIH analysis is unique in the sense that it is the most comprehensive and systematic meta-analysis looking not just at interventions of one kind but comparing, with exactly the same methodology, all factors and interventions at the same time (the Mediterranean diet, omega-3s, diabetes, statins, cognitive training, etc.).

Most major headlines around the study focused on one conclusion: that nothing can prevent Alzheimer's disease. Which, based on the study, is true. But it's not the whole truth. The meta-analysis also identified seven factors associated with both Alzheimer's disease (AD) and cognitive decline. Four of these factors were associated with increased risks: having diabetes, having the APOE e4 gene, smoking, and suffering from depression. Three other factors were associated with decreased risks: following the Mediterranean diet, being physical active, and being cognitively active. And, perhaps surprisingly in light of the of the BBC brain training study described above, cognitive training was identified as a protective factor against cognitive decline based on the highest level of evidence.

Led by the media, the main message that many people took away was: "There is nothing I can do to maintain my brain health." Which is deeply misleading, because brain health does not equal absence of Alzheimer's disease or cognitive decline, and because several manageable factors were identified to increase or decrease the risks of AD and cognitive decline. The public was thus left mostly unaware of this deeper analysis and missed the potential of the NIH meta-analysis as a great entry point to understand the effects of different interventions on brain health.

In sum, it is important to become a more critical user of the media (not to mention the Internet) when evaluating emerging scientific findings and how to apply them. We outsource many things in life – the health of your very own brain, we suggest, should not be one of them. Meaningfully integrating scientific evidence into everyday life and making good decisions in this area requires a fully engaged brain and mind.

CHAPTER HIGHLIGHTS

- Scientific findings on brain health and neuroplasticity are rapidly emerging, but only fragments of the science are presented in the media. Furthermore, what is reported is often not what is most meaningful. As a result, making sense of the scientific evidence presents a challenge.

- It is critical to complement popular media sources with independent resources, and above all with one's own informed judgment. This is especially true since not all of us have the same priorities: some focus on Alzheimer's prevention while others are more interested in maximizing functionality and quality of life now and in the near future. Meaningfully integrating scientific evidence into everyday life requires using one's most impressive tool: the brain.

INTERVIEWS

- Dr. Robert Bilder – Why and how to change the brain. Meditation is a good example.

- Dr. Alvaro Pascual-Leone – Understanding brain health to better self-monitor.

- Dr. William Reichman – Why Brain Health needs to catch up with Cardiovascular Health.

- Dr. Michael Merzenich – How Neuroplasticity will Transform Brain Health and Mental Health.

Interview with Dr. Robert Bilder – Why and how to change the brain. Meditation is a good example.

BACKGROUND

Robert M. Bilder, PhD, ABPP-CN is the Michael E. Tennenbaum Family Professor of Psychiatry and Biobehavioral Sciences at the UCLA David Geffen School of Medicine. Dr. Bilder is also the Chief of Medical Psychology-Neuropsychology at the Semel Institute for Neuroscience and Human Behavior, and directs the Tennenbaum Center for the Biology of Creativity. Dr. Bilder has been actively engaged for over 20 years in research on the neuroanatomic and neuropsychological bases of major mental illnesses.

HIGHLIGHTS:

- ⮑ Personal brain management is the next wave of human evolution.

- ⮑ Changing behavior, and thus the brain, is critical for illness prevention and better every day functioning.

- ⮑ Meditation is one of the techniques to change both brain activity and structures, and may give us unique control over attention by promoting broadening and focus.

WHY AND HOW TO CHANGE THE BRAIN

The concept of personal brain management is becoming more popular and widespread. How would you define it?

I think personal brain management is the next wave of human evolution. If we think about the great scientific revolutions, there is Copernicus who positioned earth in the universe, Darwin who positioned humans among species, and Freud, who I would argue positioned the mind inside the brain. As we learn more and more about how the brain can change its own functions, the next wave is personal brain management – using what we know about the brain to change its function.

We are doing a lot to our brains already, with drugs and psychotherapy for instance, next we will be able to modify our brain more systematically based on scientific knowledge.

Why would we want to change our brain?

Changing the brain means changing behaviors. We know now that most medical illnesses are preventable and prevention involves behavior, so being able to change our behaviors becomes crucial to preventing disease. Diseases such as cardiovascular illness, cancer and diabetes are all linked to behavior, and particularly to how we cope with stress. Other examples, such as applying sunscreen or smoking, which are related to cancer risks, also demand behavior change and particularly a better appreciation of how our current actions impact long-term outcomes.

How do we change behavior?

There is such as thing as the science of behavior change. Prochaska, a major researcher in this domain, proposes that there are a several stages of change. It starts with precontemplation (before people start thinking about a change), then moves to contemplation (when people really think about it), to action (when people are actually trying something to change) and maintenance (at least 6 months), and ends with termination (when a new behavior is in place).

Why is it so difficult to change?

A leading principle in the brain is that repetition leads to changes in the brain habit system. To reprogram the system requires effort because it requires that we inhibit prepotent, or established, response circuits.

SELF-MONITORING

To change, one needs to know what to change to start with, which implies being able to self-monitor somehow, to evaluate strengths and weaknesses and then act on this knowledge. How does one self-monitor?

Monitoring can be active. That is when we actively log information about our behaviors. Monitoring can also be passive. That is when we use devices that automatically measure our behaviors and responses. Biofeedback devices use biosensors to record all sorts of measures such as brain waves, muscles action potential, heart rate variability, respiratory rate, etc., and enable a person to *see* their own biology in a way they could never do without the sensors. The user can then work on altering the input as seen on the device by changing his or her behavior (e.g., changing breathing can alter heart rate variability and decrease stress). New tools can also help one monitoring other aspects of behavior, for instance one's mood, which allows one to understand when one is happier or sadder and whether location (home or work) or other factors play in a role. Using these monitoring devices is an input oriented way of changing a behavior. An output (or action) oriented method is to take action and repeat this action until a new habit is formed.

MEDITATION AS A TECHNIQUE TO CHANGE THE BRAIN

Can you talk about a research-based brain training technique that you think is quite effective in changing the brain?

There is a lot of interest lately in mindful awareness, brain function and health. It is well-known that Buddhist practices yield somatic control: some people manage to raise the temperature of their fingers or toes up to 17 degrees, or lower their metabolism by 64%, or decrease blood flow in the brain.

Researchers such as Richard Davidson and Antoine Lutz (2004) have shown that in very experienced meditators (that is 10,000+ hours) there is a high degree of gamma activity in the brain and greater gamma power with greater experience. Gamma waves are related to focused attention.

Are the brain activity changes triggered by meditation also observed at the structural level in the brain?

Yes. Work by Luders and colleagues in 2012 shows that in meditators there is an increased volume of the hippocampus, which is associated with memory functioning, as well as in other areas of the cortex. There is also an increased structural connectivity between regions and more gyrification (cortical folding). Interestingly, recent work by Holzel et al (2011) shows that changes can be seen very quickly: anyone doing 8 weeks of meditation can increase cortical gray matter density.

Do different types of meditation have different effect on the brain?

Focused attention meditation, where you keep your attention focused on one object, may enable us to control how much we pay attention to negative distractors and keep our attention away from these. Indeed, greater experience in this type of meditation has been shown to attenuate the activity of the amygdala in response to negative distractor sounds, presumably helping avoid distress.

Another type of meditation, open monitoring meditation (which is part of mindful awareness practice) has a different effect on the brain. It can help reduce the elaborative processing response that often follows negative distractors. This is good because it would allow us to then pay more attention to subsequent stimuli.

Interview with Dr. Alvaro Pascual-Leone – Understanding brain health to better self-monitor.

BACKGROUND

Alvaro Pascual-Leone, MD, PhD, is a Professor of Neurology at Harvard Medical School and the Director of the Berenson-Allen Center for Non-Invasive Brain Stimulation. Dr. Pascual-Leone researches the physiology of higher cognitive functions with emphasis on the study of brain plasticity in skill acquisition and recovery from injury across the lifespan. Dr. Pascual-Leone has authored more than 450 scientific papers as well as several books, and is listed as inventor in several patents.

HIGHLIGHTS:

- One main characteristic of a healthy brain is the ability to be modified – of being "plastic".

- Any activity in any one system of the brain will modify the brain in much the same way as an action will.

- Techniques to self-monitor brain health are not widely available yet. One can start by understanding what makes the brain more plastic or sustains healthy plasticity.

WHAT IS BRAIN HEALTH?

One of the goals of researchers in neuroscience is to use insights from basic science to promote healthy brain functions. Can you start by defining brain health?

A healthy brain allows us to do several things. First, having a healthy brain helps preserve cognitive ability across the lifespan. Second, it helps prevent neuropsychological and psychiatric diseases. This is crucial too because 1 in every 5 people worldwide ends up being affected by a neurological disorder across the lifespan (from development disorders such as autism or learning disabilities all the way to TBI, schizophrenia, depression, stroke, brain tumor, MS, Alzheimer's Disease). Finally having a healthy brain helps promote overall health. Indeed, our brain not only makes us capable of interacting with the outside world but also monitors our internal world which impacts our health overall. The same way a healthy body is important for a healthy brain, a healthy brain is important for a healthy body.

Can you explain the shift in the domain of disease diagnosis that is happening these days?

Nowadays we wait until a given disease manifests itself and becomes symptomatic. Then we intervene. We are quite good at diagnosing alterations of brain functions and we start to have interventions that modify diseases a little bit. A big effort today is aiming at diagnosing a disease before symptoms occur so one can modify the progression of the disease and ultimately prevent some of the symptoms. A true preventive intervention would be to intervene before any symptoms develop, when one is healthy but carry a pattern of brain activity that indicates a potential disease.

Is there one main characteristic of a healthy brain?

There are 100 billions neurons in the brain. Each neuron has about 10,000 connections (synapses) to other cells. We have 1 quintillion (10^{18}) synapses and there are 1 quintillion transactions per second between neurons. A healthy brain is thus a very complex, dynamic and efficient system. One main characteristic of such a brain is the ability of being modified, of being plastic.

The world changes very fast, too fast for genes to be able to modify our brain and make us able to cope with these changes. So nature invented plasticity, the capacity of the brain of being modified to cope with the changes in the world. We have realized that a healthy brain is a brain that has the right amount of plasticity: not too much and not too little but optimal plasticity. Plasticity changes the nature of synapses and the number of synapses in the brain. These changes can occur following any type of activity of the brain.

BRAIN NEUROPLASTICITY EXPLAINED

How does plasticity work in the brain? How fast do changes happen?

There are different steps in neuroplasticity. One is a very rapid expansion of brain matter, which can be seen in a week only (for instance when someone is learning how to play a difficult finger sequence on a piano). This expansion results from the fact that the wires that connect the neurons responsible for that learning allow more information to go through. Such expansion can be seen only during practice. When practice is stopped a shrinkage is observed. If the learning behavior is repeated over and over again, then new connections are established. In other words, the brain can accommodate more traffic and if this level of traffic is maintained it can expand the size of the road.

How is neuroplasticity influenced by genetic and environmental factors?

On one hand, people are born with more or less plasticity. For instance people with schizophrenia have certain genes that make them start with lower plasticity and quickly develop cognitive problems. Autism is the opposite. On the other hand, certain events of life can change the slope of plasticity one is in and put one at risk for developing cognitive problems. This is the case for stroke, certain diets, lack of exercise, chronic stress (particularly social stress), and illnesses like diabetes, which can all reduce neuroplasticity. Many of these factors can be manipulated, which is good news: we can intervene on our neuroplasticity.

We are in an age of great promise given the advances of neuroscience but we are in the need of debunking myths: the brain is changing all the time, some changes are good and other are not, we do have the tools to characterize these changes and thus the capacity to guide these changes for optimized functions and health.

What are the characteristics of an activity that would promote plasticity?

Chronic pain is a consequence of excessive plasticity. It is a situation where one would want to suppress plasticity so the goal is not always to promote plasticity. To promote plasticity the critical thing is it to challenge the brain to acquire new skills. For example if I am a reasonable chess player and I used to belong to a club, challenging my brain is not playing chess. For someone like me who is reading a lot and is doing a lot of intellectual activities, a good thing would be to learn to dance. For someone who does a lot of physical activities, a good thing would be to read or learn a second language. It is different for different people depending on the skills they bring to the table already. The key is to keep learning.

UNDERSTANDING THE BRAIN TO BETTER MONITOR ITS HEALTH

Thoughts and emotions can impact neuroplasticity. Can you explain how this works?

People have come to embrace the idea that interacting with the external world can change the brain (e.g., playing the piano). But what really is the case is that any activity in any one system of the brain will modify the brain in much the same way as an action will. You can modulate and modify brain connections through plastic mechanisms by repeatedly activating them. Every thought, emotion, experience, perception and action that our brain does can modify our brain. It doesn't change all at once of course but it does progressively. It thus becomes important to monitor our emotions and experiences because ultimately they can change our brain.

How can a healthy person self-monitor one's brain health?

Techniques are not widely available yet. One can understand what makes the brain more plastic or sustain healthy plasticity. We know for instance that good sleep hygiene is critical. Eating too many calories is not good for you either. Maintaining a well-balanced diet and an optimal weight is important. Regular exercise is extremely important. It doesn't need to be a lot but it needs to be regular. It appears that 15 to 30 minutes of aerobic exercise per day is needed. It is not walking from the garage to the office but going out for a run. Social interaction matters too. Social stress is bad for the brain. Interaction with a group of people who are supporting of one is important, whether this is done electronically or in person. Toxins also affect the brain dramatically: one has to be careful about what medicine one takes.

Interview with Dr. William Reichman – Why Brain Health needs to catch up with Cardiovascular Health.

BACKGROUND

In April 2008, Baycrest, a leading research institute focused on aging and brain function, received $10-million from the Ontario Government in Canada to create a groundbreaking Centre for Brain Fitness. Its stated goal was to "develop and commercialize a range of products designed to improve the brain health of aging Ontarians and others around the world".

Dr. William E. Reichman is President and CEO of Baycrest. Dr. Reichman, an internationally-known expert in geriatric mental health and dementia, is also Professor of Psychiatry on the Faculty of Medicine at the University of Toronto.

Bill, thank you for your time. Let me start by asking, given that you just spoke at the recent Consumer Electronic Show, what do you make of the growing brain fitness field?

It looks like a classic example of a very promising but still early stage field – a lot of opportunity and enthusiasm, but also a lot of product claims that are not backed by solid research. Think about the physical fitness analogy: even today, after decades of progress, you still see people buying research-based products such as treadmills but also all types of random machines they see on TV and have not been subject to any validation. Similarly, consumers today do not know what to make of growing brain fitness claims. As another speaker pointed out, for the industry to fulfill its promise, it will need to be careful with research and claims, not to end up like the nutraceuticals category.

By the way, let me recognize that the work you are doing with Sharp-Brains reports and your website is very important to offer quality information.

Thank you. Let's step back for a moment. Taking a, say, 10 year view, what is the main opportunity that technology-based brain fitness can offer to society?

First of all, let me say that I think we have an opportunity to make major progress in Brain Health in the 21st century, similar to what happened with Cardiovascular Health in the 20th, and technology will play a crucial role.

Given the rapid advances we are witnessing today in the research and technology arenas, I feel confident in saying that in less than 10 years we will have both valid and reliable assessments of cognitive functions, that will be used both by consumers at home and in a variety of health settings, and a better knowledge of what specific cognitive rehabilitative interventions may help specific groups of patients.

Quality and widely available assessments are a critical part of the puzzle. Consumers and professionals need easy-to-use, low cost assessments to measure both their needs and the impact of different interventions. Baycrest is going to take a leadership role in this area – we believe that the development of a tool equivalent to the blood pressure cuff will have great impact on brain health in the areas of prevention and treatment.

Another important component will need to be professional development and training of health professionals. What is Baycrest doing in that direction?

We are very active in knowledge exchange using modalities such as telehealth. For example, we run a Behavioral Neuroscience Rounds virtual series to share best practices with hospitals in Canada, the Middle East, and probably soon the USA too.

Tell us both about the Centre for Brain Fitness launched last year, and the Women's Brain Health Initiative you recently announced

As you know, the government of Ontario and local donors invested $20m in a new center here, housed in the Rotman Research Institute, to develop and commercialize brain fitness technologies. Baycrest has traditionally been more focused on the research than the development side, so this is a new and exciting step for us. We are now looking to hire the inaugural Director for the Centre of Brain Fitness, so let us know if you have any suggestions. We are looking for a globally recognized leader in neuroplasticity research and cognitive neurorehabilitation. As an adjunct to the Centre, we are in the process of creating a spin-off that will help identify and prioritize commercial applications of our research. You have discussed this with Veronika Litinski from MaRS Venture group who is partnering with us.

Our traditional research strengths have been cognitive assessments and cognitive rehabilitation, so it is a natural extension for us to expand our focus to include healthy aging and the needs of an aging workforce, and to investigate new platforms such as PDAs to enable people to function at the highest possible level.

The Women's Brain Health initiative was spearheaded by friends of Baycrest, active women of the baby boomer generation. They are interested in research to identify strategies and methods to prevent Alzheimer's Disease, which affects women disproportionally given their longer life expectancy and frequent status as caregivers, and also in specific gender related topics such as the impact of female hormones on brain development and function. They are raising funds to support new initiatives in women's brain health and aging at Baycrest and supporting women neuroscientists and enabling their research to be relevant and sensitive to women's brain health concerns.

A quick clarification – you mention your traditional focus on cognitive rehabilitation. Neuropsychologists have been using computerized cognitive training programs for years to support post-stroke and post-traumatic brain injury recovery, two problems that affect millions of people yet don't seem to attract enough attention given the current media theme on baby boomers and healthy aging. What is your center doing in that area?

Two of our researchers, Drs. Donald Stuss and Gordon Winocur, in collaboration with Ian Robertson of Trinity College, Dublin, recently released the main textbook in that area, titled Cognitive Neurorehabilitation, published by Cambridge University Press. You should ask them more specific questions about the present state of the field.

I will. Finally, what is the main obstacle you see today for the development of a sustainable brain fitness market that can fulfill its promise?

I'd say the lack of widely accepted standards for outcome measures. There are myriad ways to measure the impact of cognitive exercise and other lifestyle options – we can talk psychometrics, assessments of daily living, neuroimaging findings. But, there is not a consensus yet on what to measure and how.

What is one recent finding or reflection, from your own work or others', that you'd like more people of all ages to know about as they try to maintain/enhance their own brain fitness?

I continue to be impressed by the growing body of evidence that what appears good for our hearts is good for our brains. The most impressive results continue to emerge from the work supporting the vital role of an active, socially and recreationally engaged lifestyle complemented by carefully selected dietary practices, such as low fat, low sodium food choices. I am increasingly paying attention to the cognitive benefits of a structured physical fitness approach that may include a regular routine of brisk walking a few times a week. Also, emerging evidence that after retiring from work, engaging in activities such as volunteerism is helpful in maintaining strong cognitive and emotional wellbeing into later life. Other studies looking at challenging our brains through recreational activities such as playing musical instruments and taking up a second language may be effective as well. There will continue to be efforts to "exercise" and strengthen our brains through commercially developed computer based protocols and perhaps the development some day of "smart drugs" to enhance cognition. But, for the immediate future, I am focusing my attention on those lifestyle choices that most of us can fit into our daily routines and that are pleasurable.

Interview with Dr. Michael Merzenich – How neuroplasticity will transform brain health and mental health.

BACKGROUND

Dr. Michael Merzenich, Emeritus Professor at UCSF, is a leading pioneer in brain plasticity research. In the late 1980s, Dr. Merzenich was on the team that invented the cochlear implant. In 1996, he was the founding CEO of Scientific Learning Corporation (Nasdaq: SCIL), and in 2004 became co-founder and Chief Scientific Officer of Posit Science. He has been elected to the National Academy of Sciences and to the Institute of Medicine. He retired as Francis A. Sooy Professor and

Co-Director of the Keck Center for Integrative Neuroscience at the University of California at San Francisco in 2007.

Thank you very much for agreeing to participate in the inaugural SharpBrains Summit in January 2010, and for your time today. In order to contextualize the Summit's main themes, I would like to focus this interview on the likely big-picture implications during the next 5 years of your work and that of other neuroplasticity research and industry pioneers.

Thank you for inviting me. I believe the SharpBrains Summit will be very useful and stimulating, you are gathering an impressive group together.

Neuroplasticity-based Tools: The New Health & Wellness Frontier

There are many different technology-free approaches to harnessing – enabling, driving – neuroplasticity. What is the unique value that technology brings to the cognitive health table?

It's all about efficiency, scalability, personalization, and assured effectiveness. Technology supports the implementation of near-optimally-efficient brain-training strategies. Through the Internet, it enables the low-cost distribution of these new tools, anywhere out in the world. Technology also enables the personalization of brain health training, by providing simple ways to measure and address individual needs in each person's brain-health training experience. It enables assessments of your abilities that can affirm that your own brain health issues have been effectively addressed.

Of course substantial gains could also be achieved by organizing your everyday activities that grow your neurological abilities and sustain your brain health. Still, if the ordinary citizen is to have any real chance of maintaining their brain fitness, they're going to have to spend considerable time at the brain gym!

One especially important contribution of technology is the scalability that it provides for delivering brain fitness help out into the world. Think about how efficient the drug delivery system is today. Doctors prescribe drugs, insurance covers them, and there is a drug store in every neighborhood in almost every city in the world so that every patient has access to them. Once neuroplasticity-based tools and outcomes and standardized, we can envision a similar scenario. And we don't need all those drug stores, because we have the Internet!

Having said this, there are obvious obstacles. One main one, in my mind, is the lack of understanding of what these new tools can do. Cognitive training programs, for example, seem counter-intuitive to consumers and many professionals: "Why would one try to improve speed-of-processing if all one cares about is memory?" A second obvious problem is to get individuals to buy into the effort required to really change their brains for the better. That buy-in has been achieved for many individuals as it applies to their physical health, but we haven't gotten that far yet in educating the average older person that brain fitness training is an equally effortful business!

Tools for Safer Driving: Teens and Adults

Safe driving seems to be one area where the benefits are more intuitive, which may explain the significant traction.

Yes, we see great potential and interest among insurers for improving driving safety, both for seniors and teens. Appropriate cognitive training can lower at-fault accident rates. You can measure clear benefits in relatively short time frames, so it won't take long for insurers to see an economic rationale to not only offer programs at low cost or for free but to incentivize drivers to complete them. Allstate, AAA, State Farm and other insurers are beginning to realize this potential. It is important to note that typical accidents among teens and seniors are different, so that training methodologies will need to be different for different high-risk populations.

Yet, most driving safety initiatives today still focus on educating drivers, rather that training them neurologically. We measure vision, for example, but completely ignore attentional control abilities, or a driver's useful field of view. I expect this to change significantly over the next few years.

Long-term care and health insurance companies will ultimately see similar benefits, and we believe that they will follow a similar course of action to reduce general medical and neurodegenerative disease- (Mild

Cognitive Impairment and Alzheimer's and Parkinson's) related costs. In fact, many senior living communities are among the pioneers in this field.

Boomers & Beyond:
Maintaining Cognitive Vitality

Mainstream media is covering this emerging category with thousands of stories. But most coverage seems still focused on "Does it work" more than "How do we define it," "What does work mean," or "Work for whom, and for what?" Can you summarize what recent research suggests?

We have seen clear patterns in the application of our training programs, some published (like IMPACT), some unpublished, some with healthy adults, and some with people with mild cognitive impairment or early Alzheimer's Disease (AD). What we see in every case: 1) Despite one's age, brain functioning can be improved, often with pretty impressive improvement in a short-time frame and limited time invested (10 or 20 or 30 or 40 hours over a period of a few weeks up to 2 or 3 months). 2) Basic neurological abilities in 60–90 year olds that are directly subject to training (for example, processing accuracy or processing speed) can be improved to the performance level of the average 20 or 30 or 40 year old through 3–10 hours of training at that specific ability. 3) Improvements generalize to broader cognitive measures, and to indices of quality of life. 4) Improvements are sustained over time (in different controlled studies, documented at all post-training benchmarks set between 3 to 72 months after training completion).

In normal older individuals, training effects endure but that does not mean that they could not benefit from booster or refresher training — or from ongoing training designed to improve other skills and abilities that limit their older lives. Importantly, a limited controlled study in mildly cognitively impaired individuals showed that in contrast to normal individuals, their abilities declined in the post-training epoch. These folks had improved substantially with training. Even while there abilities slowly deteriorated after training, they sustained their advantages over patients who were not trained. We believe that in these higher-risk individual, continued training will probably be absolutely necessary to sustain their brain health, and, if it can be achieved (and that is completely unproven), to protect them from a progression to AD. Moreover, for both these higher-risk and normal individuals, interventions should not be thought of as one-time cure-alls. Ongoing brain fitness training shall be the way to go.

A major obstacle is that there is not enough research funding for appropriate trials to address all of these issues, especially as they apply for the mildly cognitively impaired (pre-AD) or the AD populations. We'd welcome not only more research dollars but also more FDA involvement, to help clarify the claims being made.

Next Generation Assessments

A key element for the maturity of the field will be the widespread use of objective assessments. What do you see in that area?

Unfortunately, most researchers and policy initiatives are still wedded to relatively rudimentary assessments. For example, I recently participated in meetings designed to help define a very-well-supported EU initiative on how cognitive science can contribute to drug development, in which most applied assessments and most assessments development were still paper-based. This is a major missed opportunity, given the rapidly growing development and availability of automated assessments.

I believe we will see more independent assessments but also embedded assessments. For instance, in Scientific Learning we routinely use ongoing embedded assessments and cross-referenced state test achievement scores to develop models and profiles designed to determine the regimes of neuroplasticity-based training programs that must be applied so that individual students, school sites and school districts may achieve their academic performance goals.

Implications for Medicine and Mental Health

It seems clear that neuroplasticity-related assessment and training tools will impact medicine and mental health. Where and how do you think that may happen first?

This may surprise people who haven't been following the area closely, but I believe cognitive training may well become a crucial part of the standard of care in schizophrenia over the next 3 or 4 years. With academic partners at UCSF, Yale and Konstanz University, and through the development of programs that effectively address cognitive deficits that limit this patient population, we have already designed a training program that is appropriate for evaluation in a medical-device-directed FDA trial. There is already agreement about the application of the MATRICS neurocognitive assessment battery for an FDA outcomes trial in this population, and NovaVision's FDA approval of their stroke & TBI rehab strategies provide any important FDA precedent.

The NIH has been a key enabler of the NIH Toolbox, and the MATRICS process, both to standardize assessments. What impact may these have in schizophrenia and beyond?

The FDA's adoption of MATRICS as a standard is a crucial step, because it provides a clear set of benchmarks that apply for any drug or non-drug approach to treatment. We would like to see the FDA establish similar benchmarks for all major clinical indications in neurological and psychiatric medicine. I haven't followed the Toolbox so closely, and can't really comment about its possible utility.

If we talk about wider clinical practice, we must recognize that many psychologists are attached to older forms of therapy that don't incorporate contemporary cognitive neuroscience findings, and that neurologists and psychiatrists are strongly pharmaceutically oriented, and in any event are greatly pressed for time. Perhaps clinical practice will only change once we have developed the tools necessary to help professionals monitor the brain function and training (treatment) status of the very large number of patients that might typically be under their care.

Integrating Cognition with Home Health and Medical Home Models

That's a very interesting point. How may remote monitoring and interventions happen? Is this similar to the model Cogmed uses today to deliver its working memory training via a network of clinicians?

We will probably see hybrid models emerge first. The clinician will, as usual, establish a diagnosis and initiate treatment in their office or clinic, probably with the assistance of a trained therapist. At some point, the therapy will continue at home. The therapist and the supervising clinician would be able to remotely monitor the patient's performance by the use of our Internet tools. This model, originally developed and widely applied by Scientific Learning, has also been employed by Cogmed.

Only later may full telemedicine models emerge, where perhaps a neurologist monitors the brain function of several patients using appropriate tools, and identifies potential personalized preventive interventions with red flags that call for an office (or virtual) visit.

What's Next?

This has been a fascinating conversation, and a great context to the themes we will cover in depth in the summit. What else do you think will happen over the next few years?

First, I believe we'll need to focus on public education, for people to understand the value of tools with limited face value. One important aspect of this is the need to find balance between what is fun and what has value as a cognitive enhancer which requires the activities to be very targeted, repetitive and slowly progressive – not always the most fun. People need to think fitness as much or more than games.

Second, I believe the role of providing supervision, coaching, support, will emerge to be a critical one. Think about the need for having a piano teacher, if you want to learn how to play the piano and improve over time. Technology may help fill this role, or empower and richly support real coaches who do so.

Which existing professional group is more likely to become the personal brain trainers of the future? Or will we see a new profession emerge?

Frankly, I don't know. To give you some context, at Scientific Learning we experimented with offering free access to therapists for a 2-month training. At Posit Science we first experimented with virtual coaches that many people seemed to hate, and later encouraged people who had completed the program to volunteer and coach new participants. Results were mixed. We're now exploring other possibilities.

Let me mention a few other aspects. I believe we will also see a growing number of applications in languages other than English, which will be key given growing interest in South Korea, Japan and China on aging workforce issues (until now they have been mostly focused on childhood development, using English-based programs). We will also see the programs widely available to people who may not have computers at home. For example, Posit Science recently donated software equivalent in value to $1m to the Massachusetts public library system, as a model of how wider access (in this case, to help older drivers) might be provided.

My dream in all of this is to have standardized and credible tools to train the 5–6 main neurocognitive domains for cognitive health and performance through life, coupled with the right assessments to identify one's individual needs and measure progress. For example, I'd like to know what the 10 things are that I need to fix, and where to start. Assessments could either measure the physical status of the brain, such as the degree of myelination, or measure functions over time via automated neuropsychological assessments, which is probably going to be more efficient and scalable and potentially be self-administered in a home health model.

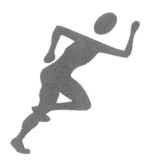

CHAPTER 3

MENS SANA IN CORPORE SANO

Now that you have been introduced to the basics of brain functioning and neuroplasticity (Chapter 1) and are equipped with the background needed to make sense of new scientific findings (Chapter 2), we can turn to the pillars of brain health and fitness, beginning with physical exercise. The existence of a relationship between the health of the body and of the mind has been appreciated for a long time. What is new is the awareness that a moderate level of aerobic exercise is a critical foundation for both that corpore sano (healthy body) and mens sana (healthy mind) – including the maintenance of the so-called executive functions that tend to decline with age. A growing body of research shows both the cognition enhancing effects of exercise as well as its potential preventative properties, which begs the question: what are the practical lifestyle implications of such findings?

HOW DOES PHYSICAL EXERCISE AFFECT THE BRAIN?

Physical exercise seems to slow, and perhaps even halt or reverse, the brain atrophy (shrinkage) that typically starts in a person's forties, especially in the frontal regions of the brain responsible for executive function. In other words, exercise (mainly aerobic exercise) can increase the brain's volume of actual neurons (referred to as "gray matter") and connections between neurons (referred to as "white matter"). This is possible because physical exercise triggers biochemical changes that spur neuroplasticity – the production of new connections between neurons and even of neurons themselves. For example, Fred Gage's work at the Salk Institute for Biological Studies has shown that exercise helps generate new brain cells, even in an aging brain. At the same time, exercise helps protect these fledgling neurons by bathing them in nerve growth factors (called "neurotrophins") which contribute to the survival, maintenance, and growth of neurons. Finally, physical exercise triggers the formation of new blood vessels (angiogenesis) in the brain.

For a while, the research supporting the multitude of effects of exercise on the brain relied on animal studies, but recent evidence obtained from human studies confirms the results from animal studies. For instance, in 2011 Eadaoin Griffin and her colleagues at the University of Dublin assessed levels of a growth factor known as brain-derived neurotrophic factor (BDNF) and memory performance of male college students before and after exercise. To establish a baseline performance, participants were first shown photos with the faces and names of strangers, and then, after a break, were shown the same photos and asked to recall the names. Next, half of the participants rode a stationary bicycle at increasing speeds until they were exhausted, while the others sat quietly for 30 minutes. Subsequently, both groups were asked to recall the names seen at the very beginning of the study, and concentration of BDNF was assessed for each participant. Interestingly, participants who performed the physical exercise saw their memory improve compared to their baseline performance, and these changes in cognitive function were accompanied by an increased concentration of BDNF. Similar results were obtained by a different team of scientists in a study with an older population (mean age: 60.5 years old): higher levels of physical activity were associated with both higher levels of G-CSF (another type of nerve growth factor) and more neuron volume (gray matter) in the prefrontal cortex, as well as with better memory performance.

Several brain imaging studies have now shown that physical exercise is accompanied by increased brain volume in humans. In one such study, researchers randomly assigned 59 older adults to either a cardiovascular exercise group or a non-aerobic exercise control group (stretching and toning exercise). Participants exercised 3 hours per week for 6 months. The researchers scanned the participants' brains before and after the training period. After 6 months, the brain volume of the aerobic exercising group increased in several areas compared to the other group. Volume increase occurred principally in frontal and temporal areas of the brain involved in executive control and memory. And in a more recent example (2009), Arthur Kramer's team looked at the relationship between physical fitness and the size of the hippocampus, a brain structure crucial for memory formation. They measured the cardio-respiratory fitness of 165 adults between 59 and 81 years of age and measured the size each individual's hippocampus. They also tested the participants' spatial reasoning. They found that the more fit people had a bigger hippocampus, and that the people who had a bigger hippocampus were also the ones who had better spatial memory.

In 2010, Kirk Erickson and his colleagues went even further and showed that levels of physical activity can predict brain volume nine years later. In this study, physical activity (how many blocks walked over one week) was first assessed. Cognitive functions of the 300 participants (age 78 on average) were assessed at the same time, as well as three to four years later, and brain scans were acquired nine years later. Greater amounts of physical activity predicted greater gray matter volume nine years later: the longer the distance people used to walk, the larger their brain volume. This effect was observed mostly in the prefrontal and temporal regions of the brain, including in the hippocampus. It was associated with a lower risk of developing dementia or mild cognitive impairment.

STAYING FIT IMPROVES COGNITION

As we have begun to see from the above studies, the biological brain changes triggered by physical exercise (e.g., increased nerve growth factor concentration and brain volume) often translate into measureable improvements in cognitive function. Recently, a review looked at 11 randomized controlled trials (RCT's) with healthy participants aged 55+ that tested the cognitive benefits of exercise. Across the studies, the exercise involved varied in intensity and duration (usually 4 months or less) but the goal was always to improve cardiorespiratory fitness. Out of the 11 studies, 8 found that the participants in the exercise training groups showed improvement in cognitive function. Another recent study involved 170 individuals age 50 and over who were randomly assigned to a physical exercise intervention (50 minutes, 3 times a week, for 24 weeks). The effect of physical exercise on cognition was modest but durable over an 18-month period.

Based on these two high-quality studies, the authors of the 2010 NIH meta-analysis concluded that physical exercise does seem to enhance cognition. The meta-analysis found that the evidence of cognitive benefits caused by physical exercise was not as strong as the evidence of cognitive benefits caused by mental exercise or challenge – but the research has been rapidly growing and shows a wide variety of benefits beyond those looked into by the NIH review, making aerobic exercise one of the lifestyle basics that we all need to address.

An astute reader might recall what we mentioned in Chapter 2 about looking carefully at the populations of participants used in a study and question if the effect of exercise on mental function appears only later in life or if it can be observed earlier. While most recent research has focused on older populations, an emerging literature suggests that physical activity and high levels of aerobic fitness during childhood may in fact enhance cognition, meaning exercise can have an impact on the brain throughout the lifespan.

In two 2010 studies by Arthur Kramer (whose interview you can find at the end of this chapter), the cognitive performance and the brains of higher-fit and lower-fit 9- and 10-year-old children were examined. In one study, fitter children did better than less fit children in a task that requires ignoring irrelevant information and attending to relevant cues. Fitter children also had larger basal ganglia than less fit children, a region known to play a key role in cognitive control (e.g., preparing, initiating, inhibiting, and switching responses). In another study, fitter children did better than less fit children in a task requiring memorization of information. Fitter children also had a larger hippocampus, a structure in the brain that is key for the formation of new memories.

These studies suggest that physical fitness in children is associated with a) better cognitive performance and b) larger brain structures (usually the ones responsible for the performance difference). The results do not show a causal relationship between physical fitness and cognitive performance. When examined in context with the results coming from the adult population however, it does seem likely that a causal effect exists.

Finally, if you are wondering what specific functions are optimized by physical exercise, the answer from the various studies appears to be: not all, but a wide range. The benefits seem to be larger for executive functions (planning, working memory, inhibition, multi-tasking, etc.). This is a key point because the brain structures supporting these functions, mainly the prefrontal cortex, are very sensitive to age-related changes.

STAYING FIT IS PREVENTIVE

Now that we've established that physical exercise can help promote cognitive functioning in the present, the natural next question is if it has any effects with regard to preventing or at least delaying cognitive decline and Alzheimer's disease onset.

In addition to the 2010 NIH meta-analysis, a number of studies looking at the factors that may help postpone the emergence of cognitive decline and/or dementia have identified physical exercise as a key factor. For instance, a large 2010 study (1000+ participants) led by Yonas Geda at the Mayo Clinic showed that any frequency of moderate exercise performed in mid-life or late life was associated with reduced odds of having Mild Cognitive Impairment. Similarly, another large study published in 2009 followed 1880 healthy 77-year old adults over 8 years, testing their cognitive functions every 1.5 years. They found that being physically active lowered the participants' risks of developing Alzheimer's disease, and further, the more active people were the less they were at risk. Note that in this population high physical activity amounted to either 1.3 hours of vigorous exercise per week, 2.4 hours of moderate exercise per week, or 4 hours of light exercise per week.

Physical exercise can also be protective against other kinds of brain-related diseases. Richard Smeyne of the Saint Jude Children's Research Hospital in Memphis found that starting an exercise program early in life was an effective way to lower the risk of developing Parkinson's disease later in life. In the same study, he found that after two months of exercise, Parkinson's patients (who demonstrate a progressive loss of dopamine neurons in a region known as the substantia nigra) had more brain cells. Higher levels of exercise were shown to be significantly more beneficial than lower amounts, although any exercise was better than none.

In sum, we can conclude that physical exercise can potentially lower risks of cognitive decline and Alzheimer's disease (AD). Note that at the time of their meta-analysis the NIH considered the level of evidence to still be low, probably because only observational studies exist so far in this area (in contrast to randomized controlled trials; see Chapter 2).

HOW MUCH EXERCISE AND WHAT KIND?

By now you are probably convinced of the many virtues of physical exercise when it comes to maintaining and improving the brain's performance. With this established, the question then becomes how much exercise, and of what kind, should a reasonable person make sure to perform in a typical weekly routine?

In terms of frequency it appears that the best regimen incorporates, at a minimum, three 30 to 60 minute sessions per week. With regard to type of exercise, the key words to remember are "aerobic" and "exercise." Physical exercise includes both aerobic exercise (also known as "cardio") and anaerobic exercise, which are distinguished by their reliance on different energy sources. Aerobic activities, such as jogging or biking, are generally light-to-moderate in intensity and longer in duration, while anaerobic activities, such as weight training, are high in intensity and shorter in duration. Of the two, aerobic exercise has been the type of activity most tested in studies, and with the more apparent benefits.

Exercise does not have to be strenuous, but it needs to be exercise. Simply going for a walk can have positive brain effects. It seems unlikely though that just walking around the house or office is enough activity. An aerobic activity will raise your heartbeat and increase your breathing rate, and this is not likely to happen if you merely walk around the block at a leisurely pace, which leads us to the second key word: exercise. Physical activity and physical exercise are different. Physical activity happens whenever we move, whether it is to lift a pencil or run a marathon. Physical exercise (e.g. swimming) refers to the effortful activity of particular parts of our bodies. While both may bring benefits, it is clearly physical exercise that helps build capacity and muscle strength. It is thus physical exercise that contributes to staying physically fit. This is the kind of exercise that also brings brain benefits.

How about non-aerobic exercise – does it have any effect on the brain? At the present, research examining this question is scarcer and less conclusive than for its aerobic counterpart. In 2009, a study showed that 12 months of once- or twice-weekly strength training improved certain executive functions (selective attention and conflict resolution). The study included 155 women aged 65-to-75 years old. Resistance training was done in 60 minute classes using a leg press and free weights. It was compared to a control balance and tone training group who used stretching, range-of-motion, basic core-strength, and balance exercises as well as relaxation techniques. The one-year follow-up study showed that the individuals who participated in the strength training exercise program had sustained cognitive benefits.

The same team of researchers recently also showed that, compared to balance and tone exercise training, twice-weekly weight training for 6 months improved executive functions in a group of women between the ages of 70 and 80 who had Mild Cognitive Impairment. In that study, the group of women who participated in the aerobic exercise training did not show any cognitive benefit. While it is encouraging to see evidence accumulate showing that strength exercise is beneficial for the brain, let's keep in mind that such evidence is still scarce compared to the numerous studies on aerobic exercise.

CHAPTER HIGHLIGHTS

- Aerobic exercise can enhance a wide variety of brain functions, especially executive functions supported by the prefrontal cortex (planning, task-switching, inhibition, etc.).

- This is possible because physical exercise triggers biochemical changes in the brain that spur neuroplasticity – the production of new connections between neurons and even of new neurons themselves.

- Exercise does not need to be strenuous – but it has to go beyond simply walking around. To be most beneficial, it needs to raise your heartbeat and increase your breathing rate.

INTERVIEWS

- Dr. Arthur Kramer – Why we need both physical and mental exercise.

- Dr. Yaakov Stern – How do physical and cognitive exercise interact?

Interview with Dr. Arthur Kramer – Why we need both physical and mental exercise.

BACKGROUND:

Dr. Arthur Kramer is a Professor in the Department of Psychology at the University of Illinois. At the University, he is part of the Campus Neuroscience Program, the Beckman Institute, and the Director of the Biomedical Imaging Center.

HIGHLIGHTS:

- ⟳ Aerobic exercise, at least thirty to sixty minutes per day, three days a week, has a positive impact on brain fitness.

- ⟳ The ideal for brain health: combine both physical and mental stimulation along with social interaction.

LIFESTYLE CHOICES TO ENHANCE BRAIN HEALTH

Let's start by trying to clarify some existing misconceptions and controversies. Based on what we know today what are the top two or three key lifestyle habits that you suggest would help someone delay Alzheimer's symptoms and improve overall brain health?

First, be active. Do physical exercise. Aerobic exercise, at least thirty to sixty minutes per day, three days a week, has been shown to have an impact in a variety of experiments. And you do not need to do something strenuous. Even walking has been shown to have this effect. There are many open questions in terms of specific types of exercise, duration, and magnitude of effect. But, as we wrote in our recent Nature Reviews Neuroscience article, there is little doubt that leading a sedentary life is bad for our cognitive health. Cardiovascular exercise seems to have a positive effect.

Second, maintain lifelong intellectual engagement. There is abundant observational research showing that doing more mentally stimulating activities reduces the risk of developing Alzheimer's symptoms.

Ideally, combine both physical and mental stimulation along with social interactions. Why not take a good walk with friends to discuss a book? We all lead very busy lives, so the more integrated and interesting our activities are, the more likely we will do them.

Great concept: a walking book club! Part of the confusion we are seeing in the marketplace is due to the search for "the magic bullet" that will work for everyone and solve all problems. We prefer to talk about the pillars of brain health (such as physical and mental exercise, stress management and a balanced nutrition) and to focus on the different priorities for each individual. Can you elaborate on what interventions seem to have a positive effect on specific cognitive abilities, for specific individuals?

Perhaps one day we will be able to recommend specific interventions for individuals based on genetic testing, for example, but we do not have a clue today. We are only beginning to understand how the environment interacts with our genome. But, I agree with the premise that there probably will not be a general solution that solves all cognitive problems, but that we need a multitude of approaches. And we cannot forget, for example, the cognitive benefits from smoking cessation, sleep, pharmacological interventions, nutrition, and social engagement.

Physical exercise tends to have rather broad effects on different forms of perception and cognition, as seen in the Colcombe and Kramer, 2003, meta-analysis published in Psychological Science.

Cognitive training also works for a multitude of perceptual and cognitive domains – but has shown little transfer beyond trained tasks. No single type of intervention is sufficient. Today there is no clear research on how those different lifestyle factors may interact. The National Institute on Aging is starting to sponsor research to address precisely this question.

Earlier you said that no brain software in particular has been shown to maintain cognition across extended periods of time. Now, didn't the ACTIVE trial five-year results show how cognitive training (computerized or not) can result in pretty durable results? For context, are there comparable controlled studies to ACTIVE where ten or more hours of physical exercise today can result in measurable (yet, incomplete) cognitive benefits five years from now?

The ACTIVE study showed a good deal of five years retention of the tasks that were trained for ten hours each, but limited transfer of training was found for other untrained tasks. It seems unlikely that significant transfer may occur with the relatively little training (e.g. ten hours in the ACTIVE study) and focused tasks that have been provided in training studies thus far.

On whether there are controlled studies similar to ACTIVE that have measured the long-term cognitive benefits of physical exercise, there are none that I know of.

What is the best way to explain the relative benefits of physical vs. cognitive exercise? It seems clear that physical exercise can help enhance neurogenesis (i.e. the creation of new neurons), yet learning and cognitive exercise contribute to the survival of those neurons by strengthening synapses, so it seems that those two "pillars" are more complementary than interchangeable

I agree. Given what we know today, I would recommend both intellectual engagement and physical exercise. However, we do know, from a multitude of animal studies, that physical exercise has a multitude of effects on brains beyond neurogenesis, including increases in various neurotransmitters, nerve growth factors, and angiogenesis (the formation of new blood vessels).

FLEXIBILITY OF SENIORS' BRAINS

Tell us more about your work with cognitive training for older adults.

We now have a study in press where we evaluate the effect of a commercially available strategy videogame on older adults' cognition (Note: this study is now published, see Basak, et al., 2008). Let me first give some context. It seems clear that, as we age, our so-called crystallized abilities remain pretty stable, whereas the so-called fluid abilities decline. One particular set of fluid abilities is called executive functions, which deal with executive control, planning, dealing with ambiguity, prioritizing, and multi-tasking. These skills are crucial to maintain independent living.

In this study, we examined whether playing a strategy-based video game can train those executive functions and improve them. We showed that playing a strategy-based videogame (Rise of Nations Gold Edition) could result in not only becoming a better videogame player but could also transfer to untrained executive functions. We saw a significant improvement in task switching, working memory, visual short-term memory, and mental rotation. And some, but more limited, benefits in inhibition and reasoning.

I can share a few details on the study: the average age of the participants was sixty-nine, and the experiment required around twenty-three hours of training time. We only included individuals who had played videogames zero hours per week for the previous two years.

That last criterion is interesting. We typically say that good "brain exercise" requires novelty, variety and challenge. So, if you take adults who are sixty-nine years old and have not played a videogame in two years, how do you know if the benefit comes from the particular videogame they played vs. just the value of dealing with a new and complex task?

That is a great question. The reality is that we do not know, since we had a "waiting list" control group. In the future perhaps we should compare different videogames or other mentally stimulating activities against each other and see what method is the most efficient. Perhaps the National Institutes of Health may be interested in funding such research.

In any case, your study reinforces an important point: older brains can, and do, learn new skills.

Yes. The rate of learning by older adults may be slower, and they may benefit from more explicit instruction and technology training; but, as a society, it is a massive waste of talent not to ensure that older adults remain active and productive.

Another recent study we conducted that is still under review is titled "Experience-Based Mitigation of Age-Related Performance Declines: Evidence from Air Traffic Control." (Note: this study is now published, see Nunes & Kramer, 2008). It deals with the question: Can age itself be an obstacle for someone to perform as an air controller? And the answer is: age itself, within the age range that we studied, is not an obstacle. Our results suggest that, given substantial accumulated experience, older adults can be quite capable of performing at high levels of proficiency on fast-paced, demanding, real-world tasks like flying planes.

The field of computerized cognitive training has the potential to work in a variety of applications beyond "healthy aging". You are obviously familiar with Daniel Gopher's work training military pilots using Space Fortress. Is your lab doing something in the area of cognitive enhancement?

Yes, I have been involved in that area of work since the late 70s, when I helped design the protocols for Space Fortress. This program indeed provides a very interesting example of real-life transfer – pilots do seem to fly better as measured by real-life instruments.

Our lab is now embarking on a five years study for the U.S. Navy to explore ways to capitalize on emerging research about brain plasticity to enhance training and performance. MIT and my lab will analyze the best training procedures to increase the efficiency and efficacy of training of individual and team performance skills, particularly those skills requiring high levels of flexibility. The results from this study will be in the public domain, so I hope they will contribute to the maturity of the field at large.

MATURITY OF THE COGNITIVE FITNESS FIELD

That is an important point. What does the field of cognitive fitness at large need to mature and become more mainstream?

We need more research, but not just any kind of research. What we need is a kind of independent "seal of approval" based on independent clinical trials. Most published research of cognitive training interventions is sponsored and/or conducted by the companies themselves. We need independent, objective and clear standards of excellence.

Interview with Dr. Yaakov Stern – How do physical exercise and cognitive exercise interact?

BACKGROUND:

Dr. Stern is the Division Leader of the Cognitive Neuroscience Division of the Sergievsky Center, and Professor of Clinical Neuropsychology at the College of Physicians and Surgeons of Columbia University, New York. He is one of the leading proponents of the cognitive reserve theory.

HIGHLIGHTS:

⮑ Exercise may impact cognition and the brain across all ages.

◌ Physical and cognitive exercise are synergistic: people may benefit more from cognitive training when they exercise, since exercise may help the brain be more receptive to this training.

SAME INTERVENTIONS FOR BOTH YOUNGER AND OLDER ADULTS?

What do you make of the recent study showing that people who stay mentally engaged beginning in childhood and remain so throughout their lives actually develop fewer amyloid plaques?

I find these results very intriguing. The concept of cognitive reserve posits that various lifetime exposures such as education, occupation and leisure activities may be related to differential susceptibility to Alzheimer's pathology once it occurs. This paper continues a new, ongoing theme that certain lifetime closures may actually impact the brain changes or pathologic findings themselves. While more work needs to be done to understand how lifetime exposures may impact the development of Alzheimer's disease pathology, it is clear that both cognitive stimulation and exercise help shape the brain throughout the lifespan. For example, animal studies indicate that both a stimulating environment and aerobic exercise are associated with neurogenesis, the growth and utilization of new neurons in the hippocampus. Thus, life events may contribute to what I have called "brain reserve," but now brain reserve is a much more fluid concept than I originally imagined.

How do these findings link to your work?

These types of observations have contributed to the design of two intervention studies that I am currently running. One of them compares people who engage in an aerobic exercise versus stretching and toning for six months. We are comparing these two forms of physical exercise to see which is more beneficial. Before and after this exercise period, the participants receive extensive cognitive evaluation and neuroimaging. The neuroimaging studies will help us understand what brain changes are associated with any cognitive improvement that we see. One unique aspect of this study is that it is enrolling younger people that have been included in previous studies. We are recruiting individuals who are 30-45 and 50-65.

What is the current understanding on what adults may need and benefit from? Are priorities and likely interventions the same when we talk about younger vs. older adults?

That is exactly what I'd like to find out. The animal studies and some studies of younger adults suggest that exercise may impact both cognition and the brain across all ages. The goal of my study is to see whether it has similar efficacy in younger and older individuals, whether the same cognitive processes are enhanced, and whether the neural basis for improvement is the same across these age groups. In the second ongoing study, we are looking at the relative benefits of physical and cognitive exercise.

HOW DO PHYSICAL AND COGNITIVE EXERCISE INTERACT?

What is the current understanding on the relative merits and shortcomings of physical and cognitive exercise? Do you see them as somehow mutually exclusive or as synergistic?

My view is that they are synergistic. It makes sense to me that any improvements in "brain reserve" would heighten the ability to develop more "cognitive reserve." To explain, we know that both exercise and cognitive stimulation affect the brain itself. For example, they both up regulate a chemical that is responsible for increased synaptic plasticity. The advantage I see to cognitive training is that it can enhance specific cognitive functions. It may be that people will be benefit more from this cognitive training when they exercise, since exercise may help the brain be more receptive to this training. To test this idea, we are running another study where participants engage in both videogames designed to enhance cognitive function (specifically, attentional allocation) and also exercise. This study is open to people aged 60 and over. I must say that this study is more demanding because it requires both visits to the gym for a week and three visits to our lab to play the video game. One unique feature of both of our studies is that we have partnered with all of the YMCA's in Manhattan, so that participants can conduct their exercise sessions in any location that is convenient to them.

Why did you select that particular videogame and not, say, Tetris or Angry Birds?

We are using the Space Fortress game because I believe that it may enhance attentional allocation and executive control. I feel that these are very important cognitive functions and enhancing them may directly impact on and improve the performance of many day-to-day activities. We are comparing the Space Fortress game with more standard computer games, since it is quite possible that they may be beneficial as well.

So, your studies will measure the impact of moving from a sedentary lifestyle to exercising at least 4 times a week. Would you expect the resulting benefit to be more or less pronounced than if someone already exercising at four times per week increases to eight times per week?

I am not sure what the answer to this is. Most exercise studies begin with people who are not regular exercisers because we believe that it will increase the chance that we can see an effect. My guess is that any increase in exercise may also be beneficial, but it would be harder to detect.

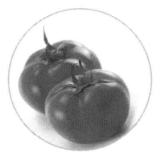

CHAPTER 4

YOU ARE WHAT YOU EAT AND DRINK (UP TO A POINT)

Exercise and nutrition both have a significant impact on our physical health. We have established that exercise also contributes to a healthy brain – but what about nutrition? Can nutrition influence how the brain works and grows? If so, what food and nutrients, if any, optimize brain health?

FOOD FOR THOUGHT

Here is a puzzle: if you inject a blue dye into the bloodstream of an animal (or a human being), what do you think will happen? As you might expect, tissues of the whole body turn blue – with the exception of the brain and the spinal cord. This is due to the presence of the (semi-permeable) blood-brain barrier (BBB) which prevents some materials in the blood, such as bacteria, from entering the brain. The BBB exists along capillaries, and consists of tights junctions around them. Cells of the barrier work to maintain a constant environment for the brain, while allowing the diffusion (movement) of essential molecules towards it.

Two such essential molecules that are allowed through the blood-brain barrier are oxygen and glucose. The brain's energy requirements are far out of proportion to the paltry 2% of the body's total weight that it represents: it receives 15% of the cardiac output, and represents 20% of total body oxygen consumption and 25% of total body glucose utilization. Looking at it another way, the brain extracts approximately 50% of oxygen and 10% of glucose from the arterial blood, incredible numbers considering its small size.

Glucose, a form of sugar, is the brain's source of fuel. Because brain cells cannot store glucose, they depend on the bloodstream to deliver it. Glucose in the blood comes mostly from carbohydrates, that is the starches and sugars that we ingest in the form of grains, fruits and vegetables, and dairy products. Complex carbohydrates (as they tend to be in natural foods) are slowly broken down and delivered to the brain. In contrast, simple carbohydrates (as in most processed and sugary foods) break apart quickly and are rapidly released in the bloodstream. This is why sugary foods that rapidly raise your blood sugar give you a quick brain boost. The effect is short-lived however, because the hormone insulin signals cells to pull the excess glucose from the bloodstream and store it for later use. Neurons are unable to store glucose however, and so they quickly deplete their fuel.

In sum, our brains need glucose to function and there are different ways to get it, with some foods (mostly natural ones) providing a better, slower, and more constant source of fuel than others (i.e., processed and high-sugar foods). This has important implications for brain performance, and establishes nutrition as another important piece of the brain fitness puzzle. At the same time, it would be a bit of an exaggeration to conclude that "we are what we eat." First of all, the blood-brain barrier doesn't allow everything to enter the brain, so not everything that is ingested can reach the brain. Second, as you will see throughout this book, many other factors influence brain functioning. Nutrition is only one part of the puzzle.

SHORT-TERM AND LONG-TERM EFFECTS OF NUTRITION

Can what we eat impact how well we function in the short-run? The answer seems to be yes. A number of studies have shown that ingesting food that provides a boost in blood glucose enhances the performance of memory and other brain functions. For instance, in a 2010 study, scientists provided healthy older adult participants who had fasted for 12 hours with either 50g of glucose or 50g of saccharin (i.e., placebo). They found that people who took the glucose were faster than people who took the placebo in a task involving attentional control.

The type of lifelong diet one follows can also impact cognition in the long-term. The Mediterranean diet has made the news quite often in recent years as a great brain-healthy diet. It typically involves a high intake of vegetables, fruit, cereals, and unsaturated fats (mostly in the form of olive oil), a low intake of dairy products, meat, and saturated fats, a moderate intake of fish, and regular but moderate alcohol consumption. Several studies have shown that the Mediterranean diet is associated with better general health as well as better brain health, with reduced risk of Alzheimer's disease and slower cognitive decline. This was confirmed by the recent NIH meta-analysis.

In 2009, Nikolaos Scarmeas, Yaakov Stern, and their colleagues from Columbia University tested whether this diet could also benefit individuals with Mild Cognitive Impairment (MCI). The term MCI applies to individuals who are in the transitional stage between normal aging and dementia of Alzheimer's (AD) or other types (some people with MCI eventually develop dementia and others do not). The study lasted approximately five years and involved 1,393 cognitively normal participants (275 of whom developed MCI during the study) and 482 participants with MCI (106 of whom developed AD during the study). Data showed that for the cognitively normal individuals, adhering to the Mediterranean diet was associated with a lower risk for developing MCI. For individuals with MCI, adhering to the Mediterranean diet was associated with a lower risk for the transition from MCI to AD. In terms of a possible mechanism, the Mediterranean diet may improve cholesterol levels, blood sugar levels and blood vessel health overall, as well as reduce inflammation (thanks to high intakes of antioxidants), factors that influence the risks for mild cognitive impairment and dementia.

So does maintaining a healthy brain require moving to live by the Mediterranean Sea? Not necessarily. One can follow such a diet anywhere in the world, and studies showing benefits from the Mediterranean diet have indeed looked at community samples from decidedly non-Mediterranean regions such as the northern part of Manhattan.

OMEGA-3 ACIDS AND ANTIOXIDANTS

While we already discussed the importance of glucose in keeping the brain running, there are a number of other molecules essential for a well-functioning brain.

The brain is a fatty organ: fats are present, for instance, in the neuron membranes and help keep them flexible. The two relevant groups of fatty acids are called omega-3s and omega-6s, which differ chemically in structure and biologically in their nutritional roles. Docosahexaenoic acid, or DHA, is the most abundant omega-3 fatty acid in cell membranes in the brain.

Our brain is dependent on dietary fat intake to get enough fatty acids. In general, a healthy diet contains a balance of the two fatty acids, omega-3s and omega-6s. In terms of the brain, recent evidence suggests that intake of omega-3 fatty acids is associated with decreased risks of cognitive decline, although no such association has been found with the risk of developing Alzheimer's disease. Unfortunately, most people in the US and Europe now get too much omega-6s and not enough omega-3s. Omega-3 fatty acids can be found in cold-water fish (such as mackerel, herring, salmon, and tuna), kiwi, and some nuts (flax seeds, walnuts). Omega-6s can be found in some seeds and nuts and the oils extracted from them (sunflower, corn, soy, and sesame oils).

Another popular nutritional factor for brain health is the intake of a group of molecules known as antioxidants that includes some common vitamins. In general, the brain is highly susceptible to a form of molecular wear and tear known as oxidative damage caused by electrically charged molecules, known as free radicals, which damage cellular DNA. Antioxidants can prevent this damage by helping to clear out free radicals. Such antioxidants are found in a variety of foods: Alpha lipoic is found in spinach, broccoli, and potatoes; Vitamin E is found in vegetable oils, nuts, and green leafy vegetables; Vitamin C in citrus fruit and several plants and vegetables. Berries are well known for their antioxidant capacity, but it is not yet clear which of their many components have an effect on cognition.

Antioxidant-rich foods have become popular for their supposed positive effects on brain function. Intake of vegetables, especially leafy green ones, and fruit to a lesser extent, has been found to be associated with both lower rates of cognitive decline and lower risks of dementia. Antioxidant supplements, however, were shown by a 2010 study to have no effects on cognitive health.

SUPPLEMENTS: GOOD, BAD, OR INEFFECTIVE?

Like many people, at some point you have probably at least considered buying nutritional supplements. It is hard to get all the important nutrients from one's diet. Supplements can be of value when a lack of a specific nutrient – a deficiency – has been identified. However, the most common purchase in this category is herbal and vitamin supplements purported to improve memory and "brainpower."

To date, no supplement has conclusively been shown to improve cognitive functioning, slow down cognitive decline, or postpone Alzheimer's disease symptoms beyond placebo effect. This was one of the key findings in the 2010 NIH meta-analysis, which reports, for instance, that there is a high level of evidence that Ginkgo biloba is not associated with reduced risk of Alzheimer's disease. Indeed, most of the recent findings associated with this well-known over-the-counter "memory-enhancing" supplement show no benefits.

For instance, a randomized 2008 trial which included 2,587 volunteers aged 75 years or older with normal cognition, showed that G biloba at 120 mg twice a day was not effective in reducing the overall incidence rate of dementia. The following year, a different study confirmed that G biloba at 120 mg twice a day did not decrease the incidence of dementia in either healthy individuals or in those with Mild Cognitive Impairment (MCI). Another randomized, double-blind, placebo-controlled clinical trial that followed 3,069 participants for an average of 6 years concluded that the use of Ginkgo, 120 mg twice daily, did not result in less cognitive decline in older adults (72-96 years old) regardless of whether they had normal cognition or MCI.

In the same way, there is a good amount of evidence showing that vitamins B12, E, C, and beta carotene have no effect on the risks of Alzheimer's and cognitive decline. Folic acid is the only supplement that appears to potentially decrease the risk of Alzheimer's, but it is not associated with a decreased risk of cognitive decline.

An additional reason to be cautious with herbal supplements is the fact that some such products have been shown to counteract the effects of prescription and over-the-counter medications. For example, in 2001, Stephen Piscitelli and his colleagues at the National Institute of Health showed a significant drug interaction between St. John's wort (hypericum perforatum), an herbal product sold as a dietary supplement, and Indinavir, a protease inhibitor used to treat HIV infection. The herb can also cause negative interactions with cancer chemotherapeutic drugs and with birth control drugs.

DOES WHAT WE DRINK AFFECT THE BRAIN?

Two kinds of beverages have been repeatedly investigated as far as brain health is concerned: coffee and alcohol.

Caffeine belongs to a chemical group called the xanthines, and it has the short-term effect of speeding neurons up. This increased neuronal activity triggers the release of the hormone adrenaline, which affects your body in several ways: your heartbeat increases, your blood pressure rises, your breathing tubes open up, and sugar is released into the bloodstream for extra energy. So, in moderate doses (a few cups a day), caffeine can increase alertness.

But is there a sustained, lifetime, benefit or harm from drinking coffee regularly? The answer, so far, contains both good news and bad news for coffee drinkers. The good news is that most of the long-term results are more positive than negative, so no clear harm seems to occur. The bad news is that results are not consistent as to whether caffeine has any beneficial effects on general brain function, in either the short-term or in delaying age-related decline or dementia over the long-term.

Another molecule that acts on the brain is alcohol. It is well known that excessive consumption of alcohol damages the brain. The effect of moderate consumption is less clear. The recent NIH meta-analysis reported that light-to-moderate drinkers may have a lower risk of cognitive decline, but the results are not consistent. Although studies show obvious differences (for instance the definition for light to moderate drinker varies across the studies from 1 to 2 drinks per week as a minimum to 13 to 28 drinks per week as a maximum), there seems to be no clear explanation for these inconsistencies. Results are more consistent however when the impact of alcohol consumption on the risks of Alzheimer's disease (AD) is considered. The same meta-analysis concludes that light-to-moderate drinkers (male and female) have a lower risk of AD compared to non-drinkers. Of note, since most studies look at alcohol consumption later in life, it is not clear whether it is late-life consumption that has an effect on risk of dementia or consumption throughout adulthood.

While we still do not fully understand how alcohol may cause these long-term effects, the most plausible explanation is that alcohol lowers rates of cardiovascular diseases. This is triggered by alcohol-induced elevations in HDL cholesterol and reduction in factors that can cause thrombosis (blood clotting). Moderate alcohol intake could thus help preserve the brain's vascular system and prevent strokes, resulting in better cognition and lower risk of dementia. Of note, people who continue to drink alcohol late in life also tend to be healthier in general, which could be a confounding factor explaining why alcohol appears to lower the risk of developing dementia.

TWO HEALTH-RELATED FACTORS THAT MATTER: DIABETES AND SMOKING

As pointed out by Larry McCleary (whose interview you can find at the end of this chapter), few people are aware that one of the earliest signs of impending dementia is a decrease in the ability of the brain to use glucose efficiently. As such a dysfunction is at the core of diabetes, some neuroscientists refer to Alzheimer's disease as Type 3 Diabetes. The recent NIH extensive meta-analysis shows that diabetes is associated with both higher risk of cognitive decline and higher risk of developing Alzheimer's disease. Diabetes is thus a high risk factor for cognitive dysfunction. This may be because microvascular disease (affecting very small scale blood vessels) is the hallmark of poor glyceamic control in people with diabetes. Another possibility is that hyperglycaemia (high blood sugar), which can alter blood flow in the brain, may also impair cognition. This knowledge is important as the awareness that diabetes impacts cognition can empower patients and may allow them to try to compensate by choosing lifestyles or targeted interventions known to enhance cognition and/or reduce risks of cognitive decline and dementia.

What about cigarette smoking? Current smokers are clearly at greater risk of Alzheimer's disease, and they show greater cognitive decline compared to people who have never smoked. Quitting smoking may help though: former smokers may show a greater yearly decline than those who never smoked, but they do not appear to be at increased risk of Alzheimer's disease, unlike current smokers. Note that these results refer to smoking and the effects can probably be attributed to tobacco, while the effects of nicotine itself may be different. Indeed some studies suggest that nicotine may boost some cognitive functions (attention, processing speed and memory), although strong evidence is still lacking.

OBESITY AND COGNITION

The nature of the relationship between weight and cognition is not clear at this time. The few studies that examined the association between weight and cognitive decline are inconclusive. Contradictory results are also reported by studies looking at the association between obesity and risks of Alzheimer's disease: some show increased risks and others decreased risks. It may be the case that the effect of weight on cognition is small. Another factor may be that the age at which people are obese matters. Indeed a study suggests that weight does not consistently predict dementia risks across the lifespan: a high body mass index could indicate higher risk of dementia early on, but later in life it may indicate lower risk. One explanation for such a finding is that, as these associations do not imply a causal relationship, decreasing weight could be an early sign of dementia (instead of a risk factor).

A recent review of 38 studies reports no association between mid-life obesity and dementia in later life, but suggests that there may nonetheless be a relationship between obesity and cognition. Obese individuals tend to have lower performance in planning, reasoning and problem solving (so-called executive functions). This may have an impact on eating behavior and exacerbate weight gain. Such gain may in turn have a negative influence on the brain via biological mechanisms (such as inflammation, elevated lipids, and/or insulin resistance). Note that whether obesity is a cause or a consequence of these cognitive deficits is unclear, which means that the safest and smartest course of action is to take care of both nutrition and cognition, not just one or the other. This also reinforces a major theme of this book: it makes more sense to effectively address the basics than to count on "magic pill" solutions.

CHAPTER HIGHLIGHTS

◌ The brain constitutes only 2% of total body weight but accounts for 25% of the total body glucose utilization. Its energy needs are great, which is part of the reason why what we ingest can affect how well we function cognitively.

◌ The effects of nutrition can be short-term (such as a surge of energy and a resulting brain boost) but also long-term. For instance, high adherence to the Mediterranean Diet (high intakes of vegetables, fruits, cereals, moderate intake of fish and alcohol and low intakes of dairy products, meat) helps reduce risks of cognitive decline and dementia.

◌ Of note, no nutritional supplement has been shown to effectively and safely improve cognition in healthy individuals: overall diet is what matters.

INTERVIEWS

⋑ Dr. Larry McCleary – A multi-pronged approach to brain health.

Interview with Dr. Larry McCleary –
A multi-pronged approach to brain health.

BACKGROUND:

Dr. Larry McCleary is a former acting Chief of Pediatric Neurosurgery at Denver Children's Hospital and author of *The Brain Trust Program* (2007).

HIGHLIGHTS:

⋑ Brain health requires a holistic approach involving appropriate nutrition, stimulating brain activities, physical activities, and stress reduction.

⋑ No matter one's brain status or age, there is much that can be done to improve brain functions.

BRAIN HEALTH IS AVAILABLE TO EVERYONE

As a neurosurgeon, how did you develop an interest in brain health public education?

For two reasons: I am a Baby Boomer and am trying to maximize my own brain health. Also, there is a great deal of exciting research documenting how we can be proactive in this regard. This information needs to be disseminated and I would like to help in this process.

And what is the single most important brain-related idea or concept that you would like every person in the planet to fully understand?

The most important take home message about brain health is that we now know that no matter what your brain status or age, there is much you can do to significantly improve brain functions and slow brain aging. Based on emerging information, what is especially nice is the fact that unlike many things in life our brain health is largely under own control.

NOURISHING OUR BRAINS

What are the most important elements to nourish our brains as we age?

I approach this question much like how an athlete prepares for a competition. Professional athletes use a holistic approach. This is also what a healthy brain requires. It should not be surprising that "what is good for the body is good for the brain." That is how our bodies and brains evolved.

Hence what I believe are valuable components of a well-rounded approach to brain health are appropriate nutrition, stimulating brain activities, physical activities, and stress reduction.

How can we nourish our brains?

The major fuel the brain consumes is glucose. The earliest sign of impending dementia and Alzheimer Disease (AD) is a decrease in the ability of the brain to use glucose efficiently. Based on this observation, some neuroscientists are referring to AD as Type 3 diabetes because of the inability to appropriately use glucose in that disorder. This makes sense because people with diabetes have a four-fold increase in AD.

The brain is a fatty organ. The most important fats are those in the nerve cell membranes whose presence keeps them flexible. These are the long chain omega-3 fatty acid molecules found in fatty, cold-water fish and arachidonic acid (a long chain omega-6 fatty acid). These are both delicate fats and as such can oxidize easily (meaning they can become rancid). Thus, we should include additional dietary components that provide free radical fighting activity to protect them against oxidation.

Based on these observations, I recommend a diet containing fatty fish, veggies and salads, non-starchy fruits (like berries) – that are high in free radical fighting compounds – and nuts.

PILLARS OF BRAIN HEALTH

What is the value of stimulating brain activity?

To increase neuroplasticity (the continual ability of the brain to "rewire" itself) and neurogenesis (the formation of new nerve cells), brain stimulation is vital. All types count including schoolwork, occupational endeavors, leisure activities and formal brain training. The key in any activity is to include novelty (to encourage thinking outside the box), challenge and variety.

And physical activity?

Exercise delivers additional blood and oxygen to the brain. Yet, it does so much more. It actually causes alterations in the nerve cells. They produce more neurotrophins, which are compounds that increase the formation of new nerve cells and enhance their connectivity. They also make the neurons we have more resistant to the aging process. I recommend cross-training your brain by starting with a good aerobic program and mixing in resistance (weight training) exercise and speed and agility components such as jumping rope, playing ping-pong, gymnastics and various balance drills.

How does stress reduction relate?

Chronic, unremitting stress kills neurons. This is especially detrimental to memory function. So include a component of stress reduction in your approach to optimal brain health and make sure to get plenty of sleep.

Also, be aware of the side effects of some medications. There are medications that lower the level of important brain nutrients in the body such as B vitamins and coenzyme Q10. Check with your doctor to screen for these. There are also many common medicines (many OTC) that have anti-cholinergic activities. These can impair the function of one of the most important memory neurotransmitters in the brain – acetylcholine.

ADVICE FOR HEALTH PROFESSIONALS

What brain health-related information or practices would you suggest to other doctors and health professionals, both for themselves and for the patients they see?

They should counsel their patients on tips for brain health such as those listed above in much the same way they discuss cardiac risk factors and how to address them.

What is one recent finding or reflection, from your own work or others', that you'd like more people of all ages to know about as they try to maintain/enhance their own brain fitness?

A recent and pivotal observation that should be publicized was recently published in the British Medical Journal on January 5, 2012. Life expectancy continues to increase and understanding cognitive aging is one of the most pressing issues of our time. As mentioned in the BMJ article, the draft fifth edition of the Diagnostic and Statistical Manual of Mental Disorders (www.dsm5.org) suggests replacing dementia with "major" and "minor neurocognitive disorder," a change that is likely to focus attention on the better understanding of age on cognition. This showcases the identification of the determinants of cognitive decline and the extent to which functional cognitive trajectories are able to be modified.

This is particularly important because therapeutics for dementing illnesses have provided little symptomatic benefit and essentially no reversal of the underlying causative factors of the disease. Based on these salient observations, there is a major effort to develop diagnostic tools that identify those at risk earlier in the course of the disorder and to provide an earlier therapeutic window — allegedly before significant brain tissue loss has occurred.

Based on previous research, no significant degree of cognitive decline was felt to be present prior to age 60. The BMJ article presents compelling findings that identify progressive cognitive falloff as early as age 45! Other evidence suggests the importance of healthy lifestyles and cardiovascular risk factors in dementia. And since most researchers believe that adverse cognitive outcomes such as dementia are thought to be the result of long term processes spanning 20 – 30 years, the lower age threshold for cognitive deterioration identified in the BMJ article suggests that initiating a brain health program early in life — certainly earlier than age 60 — is warranted.

You only live one life and only have one brain. This information should be a wake-up call to start early to preserve and protect it.

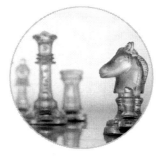

CHAPTER 5

OH, THE PLACES YOU'LL GO!

We have all heard people say things like "use it or lose it" in various contexts. The phrase is now often applied to the brain and its abilities, and the basic idea makes intuitive sense, especially in light of our capacity for lifelong plasticity. Less common however is a detailed discussion of the relative effectiveness of different forms of "mental exercise." Are all ways to "use it" equally valuable?

STRUCTURAL BENEFITS OF MENTAL CHALLENGE

As we saw in Chapter 1, the "cells that fire together, wire together" principle rules brain development. Neurons that are frequently active at the same time become closely associated and connected, or "wired." The more often neurons fire together, the stronger the connections become, and new connections can of course be created – which is especially important to help newly created neurons "hook into" pre-existing networks. Conversely, the less a network of neurons is activated, the weaker the connections become and the more likely the individual neurons are to die. In other words, using neuronal networks reinforces connections and elicits the growth of new connections. But, as we will see, not all kinds of mental activity have the same impact on neural networks.

Mental activity versus mental challenge

Mental activity takes place every waking moment, whether you are daydreaming, reading a book, or learning a new language. Our brains are even active when we rest. It would be a mistake, however, to assume that this baseline activity is sufficient to generate neuroplastic changes in the same way that actual mental exertion does, just as it is a mistake to ignore the differences between physical activity and physical exercise. Physical activity occurs whenever you perform any action that involves moving your body, whether it is brushing your teeth or playing soccer. Physical exercise (e.g. playing basketball) refers to the subset of physical activities that are effortful and challenge particular parts and muscles of our bodies. While both physical activity and physical exercise may bring benefits, it is the latter that helps build capacity and muscular strength, contributing to staying fit. Similarly, one needs to go beyond mere mental activity to generate significant change in the brain. Learning and mastering new skills is what builds and strengthens neural connections, and we can stimulate learning by exposing ourselves to activities that challenge the routine and the familiar.

A 2006 study conducted by Susan Landau and Mark D'Esposito at the University of California, Berkeley illustrates this well. Participants were taught a finger sequence to play on the piano. At the same time their brain activity was recorded. Motor areas primarily engaged by the task showed great activity while the sequence was learned. Importantly, after the sequence was learned, the activity decreased. The change in activity directly reflects changes at the level of the connections between neurons, showing an improvement in neuronal efficiency. As learning progresses, routine is established and neurons do not need to work as hard.

Trying to learn new activities is never easy. It means expending effort and getting out of your comfort zone – which is one of the reasons why we devote Chapter 7 to managing stress and building resilience. Engaging in a challenging new activity often requires confronting fears of failure and of change. Then comes the matter of deciding what level

The SharpBrains Guide to Brain Fitness

of challenge is right. A challenging activity for one person could be an impossible task for somebody else and a trifle for a third individual. The best judge of whether an activity is challenging is the person who is trying to tackle it. Whatever the activity, the goal is to be exposed to novelty and increasing levels of challenge, so that the task never becomes too easy or routine.

In other words, perhaps the single best piece of advice is to protect throughout life the beautiful spirit of curiosity and wonder espoused in the classic children's book, "Oh, the Places You'll Go!"

Challenge but also variety

Notice the word "places" – not a single "place." Many people feel that they are doing the best for their brain after having completed their daily "use it or lose it" routine, such as a crossword or Sudoku puzzle. But crossword puzzles challenge a very narrow range of cognitive skills, and evidence showing direct benefits is scarce. A 1999 study showed that increased experience in doing crossword puzzles does not modify the effect of age on cognition, as measured through tasks requiring vocabulary and reasoning. Crossword puzzles can be a stimulating activity, but they do not, beyond those first dozen or so puzzles, present substantial challenge or variety.

Given the range and interconnectedness of our brain functions, a variety of challenging activities are needed to stimulate the whole brain. Recent (2006) recommendations made by a panel of experts reviewing a poll by the American Society on Aging stated: "A single activity, no matter how challenging, is not sufficient to sustain the kind of mental acuity that virtually everyone can achieve." Even if one's goal is to improve memory functions, achieving such improvement requires stimulating other brain functions, such as attention and concentration.

Excessive specialization is not the best strategy for maintaining long-term brain health. A stock and bond trader may thus want to try an artistic activity to stimulate skills that he or she rarely uses otherwise, while an artist who has never before played videogames may want to try one of the so-called Massive Multi-Player Online Videogames, which involve planning and implementing complex strategies.

INVEST IN YOUR COGNITIVE OR BRAIN RESERVE

Not only are novelty, challenge, and variety important for improving brain fitness and ability, but research has clearly shown that frequent participation in mentally stimulating activities can successfully delay (although not prevent) cognitive decline and symptoms of Alzheimer's disease by increasing something called the cognitive (or brain) reserve.

The research behind cognitive reserve shows that it is possible to build up the brain's resilience and efficiency over time, making it better equipped to suffer neuronal damage and to delay the onset of dementia symptoms. It stems from the repeated observation that the relationship between clinical symptoms and actual brain pathology is not a direct one. For example, in 1989 Robert Katzman and his colleagues described 10 cases of cognitively normal older adults who, at death, were discovered to have advanced Alzheimer's disease pathology in their brains. The researchers hypothesized that these individuals did not show symptoms of Alzheimer's because they had more neurons, more connections between them, and more glial cells. The idea is that having a larger "reserve" of neurons and abilities can offset the losses caused by Alzheimer's and other dementias, so that a person, on average, can tolerate progressive brain pathology (including Alzheimer's plaques and tangles) without demonstrating cognitive failure.

Even more promising, one of the latest studies on the topic showed that lifelong brain stimulation lowers levels of the protein responsible for the brain plaques that constitute a hallmark of Alzheimer's disease. The 2012 study assessed the association between cognitively engaging activities (reading books or newspapers, writing letters or emails, going to the library, and playing games) and the accumulation of beta-amyloid protein in the brain. How often participants (healthy older adults, adults with Alzheimer's, and young controls) engaged in these activities was assessed at five age periods: 6, 12, 18, and 40 years and at the current age. The main finding of the study was that greater participation in mentally stimulating activities, especially in early and middle life, was associated with lower accumulation of beta-amyloid in the brain. Older participants who engaged the most in stimulating activities showed levels of protein accumulation similar to those present in the brains of young participants. In contrast, older participants who engaged the least in stimulating activities showed levels of protein accumulation similar to those present in the brains of the patients with Alzheimer's disease.

LIFELONG EFFECTS OF COGNITIVE EXERCISE

A study published in 2010 triggered a wave of puzzling headlines claiming that "Doing Puzzles Might Speed Up Dementia" or that "Brain Exercise May Worsen Existing Alzheimer's."

The study followed more than 2,000 individuals, age 65 and over, for 12 years. All participants were free of dementia or mild cognitive impairment when the study commenced. The frequency of their participation in cognitive engaging activities was first assessed in the beginning of the study. Six years later clinical evaluation was conducted to determine who was still highly functioning, who was suffering from mild cognitive impairment and who had Alzheimer's disease. The rate of cognitive decline of individuals in these three categories was then assessed over an average of 6 years. This study was different from the previous ones showing that healthy people who are cognitively active have lower risks of developing dementia for one major reason: it assessed the fate of cognitively active individuals who had been diagnosed with dementia.

The results of the study showed two trends for people with high cognitive activity scores. First, when these people had no cognitive impairment, they declined more slowly than individuals who were less cognitively active in the past. Second, once these people were diagnosed with dementia they showed compressed rates of decline.

This means that, after diagnosis, compared to less cognitively active people, they declined faster. This is illustrated in Figure 4.

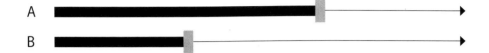

Figure 4. This is a simple graphic representation of the results, shown on a time line. Individuals cognitively active before the study began (A) are represented by the top line. Individuals less cognitively active before the study began (B) are represented by the bottom line. The thick line represents the time that individuals live without impairment. The red mark represents Alzheimer's diagnosis. The thin line represents the time that individuals live with dementia.

Such results confirm that engaging in stimulating activities helps build brain reserve. As a consequence, if dementia is not present, normal cognitive decline is slower (compared to the decline seen in less active individuals). The results also show that if dementia is present, the brain can tolerate more dementia-related pathology and still function normally, thus effectively postponing the onset of dementia. However, the brain can only tolerate pathology to a certain point. Cognitively active people who are diagnosed with dementia have reached a threshold at which it becomes very hard to function normally: they have more pathology in the brain than less active people when they are diagnosed with dementia. As a consequence, they will decline faster, which means that they will live less time with the disease. In sum, mentally stimulating activities do not accelerate dementia, they help postpone its onset. As the author puts it, the results can be explained in terms of "buying extra-time living as a highly functional individual and spending less time living with dementia."

A very different conclusion than what you might have gathered from the headlines.

In short, cognitive exercise is a key pillar for lifelong brain fitness. Mental stimulation that incorporates novelty, challenge, and variety, can improve brain functioning in the here-and-now, as well as increase brain reserve and thereby enable the brain to function normally for longer, even in the presence of a neurological disease. The real questions are: what types of cognitive exercise seem to help and what are ways to incorporate them into one's life?

EDUCATION AND OCCUPATION ARE PROTECTIVE

Research on cognitive reserve finds that the more education a person has, the less he or she tends to suffer from age-related decline. High levels of education have also been repeatedly associated with lower risk levels for Alzheimer's disease. The 2010 NIH meta-analysis confirmed that overall, education has a protective effect on the brain, especially by reducing risks of Alzheimer's disease.

How does education affect the brain? First, learning changes the brain, and so spending more time learning as children, adolescents, and adults likely triggers more changes – that is, the creation of more connections and even new neurons. Another way education could affect the brain is by the impact it has on the type of job one has. As well-educated people are more likely to have mentally stimulating jobs, it is possible that the effect of education is related to the effects of intellectual stimulation not just early in life but throughout life, through decades of work over the course of a career. And the effects of one's job seem to last even after retirement. In one study, researchers followed a large sample of participants for many years and showed that as the adults in the study grew older, the level of complexity of their past work continued to affect their level of intellectual functioning. Conversely, a 2010 study looking at the United States, England, and 11 other European countries found that the earlier people retire, the more quickly their memory declines.

LEISURE ACTIVITIES TO BUILD BRAIN RESERVE

In most studies on cognitive and brain reserve, intellectual engagement is assessed by looking at how often people participate in stimulating leisure activities. In a 2001 study conducted by Yaakov Stern at

Columbia University, individuals with the highest level of stimulating leisure activities presented thirty-eight percent less risk (controlling for other factors) of developing Alzheimer's symptoms. For each additional type of activity, the risks were reduced by eight percent.

In terms of specifics, the activities most often studied in research are: reading (books or newspapers), writing (letters or emails), playing board or card games, doing crosswords and other puzzles, and participating in organized group discussions.

The only leisure activity that has been associated with reduced brain function is watching television. This has been shown, for instance, by one study which followed more than 5,000 individuals, aged 55 years and older, for 5 years. As the years went by, some of the individuals showed cognitive impairment (at a rate of 2.3% per year). Playing board games and reading was found to be associated with a reduced risk of cognitive impairment. In contrast, watching television was associated with increased risks.

Most leisure activities have the potential to build brain reserve. As outlined above, their potential will be greater if they present a level of novelty and challenge for the person engaging in them. As Dr. Yaakov Stern puts it: "What is very exciting is that, no matter one's age, education and occupation, our level of participation in leisure activities has a significant and cumulative effect. A key message here is that different activities have independent, synergistic effects. This means that the more things you do and the earlier you start, the better. But you are never stuck. It is better to start late than never." (Find more from Dr. Stern in his interview at the end of this chapter).

Musical training

Playing an instrument often comes to mind when people are asked about the kind of activity they think is good for brain health. The reason behind this is that musicians' brains are often used as models of neuroplasticity: numerous studies have shown that musical training can change the brain. Musicians have larger brain volume in areas that are important for playing an instrument: motor, auditory and visuospatial regions. But musical training can also benefit the brain beyond technical musical ability. Specifically, musicians may have an advantage for processing speech in challenging listening environments compared with non-musicians.

Playing an instrument, even as an amateur, may also protect the brain later on against dementia-related damage. In 2011, researchers had 70 people age 60 to 83 perform a variety of tests to measure both visuospatial memory and the brain's ability to adapt to new information. Participants who had engaged in musical activity for 10 years or longer scored substantially better than those with no musical activity in their past. This was true whether the musicians were currently involved in making music or not.

Learning a new language

Another kind of stimulating activity backed-up by evidence is learning and practicing a new language. Being bilingual triggers a variety of beneficial plastic changes in the brain. Research led by Ellen Bialystok shows that speaking more than one language enhances executive functions and helps build cognitive reserve and protect against the risks of cognitive decline and Alzheimer's. For instance, in a 2007 study looking at 184 patients with dementia, 51% of whom spoke 2 languages, bilinguals showed signs of dementia 4 years later than monolinguals.

Why would bilingualism be protective? A potential explanation is that bilinguals often have to choose which language to use and which to suppress. This provides constant exercise for the frontal lobes, the area of the brain right behind the forehead that focuses our attention, helps us ignore distractions, and makes decisions. Indeed, evidence suggests that bilinguals are faster and more efficient in tasks where executive functions (supported by the frontal lobes) are required.

How about video games?

When it comes to the effects of video games on their players, it is much more common to hear about potential negatives like increases in aggression and antisocial behavior than about improvements in brain function. It appears though that while these negative effects may possibly occur with extremely violent video games and for very specific groups of players, it doesn't seem to be the case for most games or for most players. Additionally, studies are showing that specific types of video games can, in fact, optimize specific brain functions.

Action video games: Playing action video games can boost performance in a variety of sensory, perceptual, and attentional tasks, even in tasks very different from the ones involved in the game played. Daphne Bavelier and her team have conducted many studies in which they used action video games as brain training tools. They have shown that training for as little as ten hours on action video games (such as Medal of Honor, Call of Duty, and Unreal Tournament) can lead to enhancements in the ability to spread attention around the visual field, to keep track of multiple moving objects, and to pick out relevant information from a rapid sequence of visual events. Action videogame training can also positively affect more basic aspects of vision, such as the ability to resolve small details or see faint patterns. Dr. Bavelier argues that a large portion of the population could benefit from such enhancements, since excellent vision and visual attention are important skills for many professions (military personnel, taxi drivers, firefighters, athletes, etc.).

Rise of Nations (strategy game): It also appears that certain strategy video games can improve working memory. A 2008 study by Arthur Kramer and his colleagues involving participants age 60 and older compared a group who were asked to play a role-playing strategy computer game called Rise of Nations with a control group. The goal of the game is to build an empire, and players must build cities, sustain a population, build and maintain a military, and defeat other players. Assessments conducted before, during, and after the video game training showed that, as a group, the game-players showed significant improvements in their ability to switch between tasks as compared to the control group. Both their working memory and reasoning ability also showed notable improvement.

Prosocial games: In an intriguing 2010 study, researchers tested whether playing games that involve concern for the welfare of others and empathetic action would enhance players' real life social behavior. Participants played either a prosocial game, Lemmings, which asks players to ensure the safety of a group of creatures, or a neutral game such as Tetris. Then the researchers placed the participants in situations where they had the opportunity to help others, ranging from low-risk situations (e.g., seeing a dropped cup of pencils) to high-risk ones (e.g., witnessing an angry ex-boyfriend harass an experimenter). The results suggested that playing the prosocial game boosted the altruism of the players: these participants were much more likely to help in both types of situations than were those who had played a neutral game.

Nintendo DS Brain Age: There is very limited evidence so far that playing Nintendo's Brain Age can boost brain functions. A recent very small study suggested that playing Brain Age (in contrast to playing Tetris) for four weeks improved executive functions and processing speed in the elderly. Of note, the study was not run in a completely independent manner, as Ryuta Kawashima (the inventor of the game) was one of the co-authors. Another recent study reported an increase in performance in a working memory task after a 6-week period during which participants (74 years old on average) played Brain Age 2-3 times a week. A few methodological questions arise with this study though: in addition to the small number of participants (41 total), the authors report that how often the participants played was not controlled, and thus very variable. Finally, players were compared to a group of people who did nothing in particular during the intervention period, which is a poor scientific control.

In short, playing some types of mainstream video games can enhance brain function, suggesting that they constitute rather stimulating activities. No conclusive study so far has shown that playing video games triggers any kind of long-term protective effect, which is why they were not explicitly identified as protective in the 2010 NIH meta-analysis. Having said that, they can be an excellent vehicle for novelty, variety and challenge, and a rather stimulating alternative to crossword puzzle number one million and one.

CHAPTER HIGHLIGHTS

- ➲ "Use It or Lose It" is not about doing one more crossword puzzle, it is about "stretching" our mental capacity often and in new, varied, and challenging ways.

- ➲ Maintaining functionality longer in healthy individuals is as important as preventing Alzheimer's pathology.

- ➲ Lifelong participation in cognitively engaging activities results in delayed cognitive decline in healthy individuals and in spending less time living with dementia in people diagnosed with Alzheimer's disease.

INTERVIEWS

- ➲ Dr. Yaakov Stern – The connection between building a cognitive reserve and delaying Alzheimer's symptoms.

- ➲ Dr. Elizabeth Zelinski – Healthy aging and cognitive enhancement.

Interview with Dr. Yaakov Stern – The connection between building a cognitive reserve and delaying Alzheimer's symptoms.

BACKGROUND:

Dr. Stern is the Division Leader of the Cognitive Neuroscience Division of the Sergievsky Center, and Professor of Clinical Neuropsychology at the College of Physicians and Surgeons of Columbia University, New York.

He is one of the leading proponents of the cognitive reserve theory, which aims to explain why some individuals with Alzheimer's pathology (accumulation of plaques and tangles in their brains) can maintain normal lives until they die, while others with the same amount of plaques and tangles display the severe symptoms we associate with Alzheimer's Disease.

HIGHLIGHTS:

- A lifetime of engaging activities has a positive cumulative effect: Lifetime factors such as education, occupation, and activities, have a major influence on how we age. The more activities we do throughout our lives, the better.

- Stimulating activities, ideally combining physical exercise, learning, and social interaction, help build a cognitive reserve to protect us. The earlier we start building our reserve, the better; but it is never too late to start.

DEFINING THE COGNITIVE RESERVE

The implications of your research are astounding, presenting major implications across sectors and age groups. What has been the most unexpected reaction you have received so far?

I was pretty surprised when, years ago, a reporter from Seventeen magazine requested an interview. I was really curious to learn why she felt that her readers would be interested in studies about dementia. What she told me showed a deep understanding and insight: she wanted to motivate children to stay in school and not drop out. She understood that early social interventions could be very powerful for building a reserve and preventing dementia.

Fast forward 60 or so years from high-school. Suppose that two people A and B both technically have Alzheimer's (plaques and tangles appear in the brain), but only A is showing the disease symptoms. What may explain this discrepancy?

Individuals who lead mentally stimulating lives, through education, occupation and leisure activities, have reduced risk of developing Alzheimer's. Studies suggest that they have thirty-five to forty percent less risk of manifesting the disease. The pathology will still occur, but they are able to cope with it better. Some will not ever be diagnosed with Alzheimer's because they will not present any symptoms. In studies that follow healthy elders over time and then study their brains through autopsies, up to twenty percent of people who did not present any significant problem in their daily lives have full blown Alzheimer's pathology in their brains.

What is going on in the brain to provide that level of protection?

There are two ideas that are complementary. One idea (called brain reserve by researchers) postulates that some individuals have a greater number of neurons and synapses, and that somehow those extra structures provide a level of protection. In a sense, they have more "hardware", providing a passive protection against the attacks of Alzheimer's.

The other theory (called cognitive reserve) emphasizes the building of new capabilities, how people can perform tasks better through practice, and how these skills become so well learned that they are not easy to unlearn. It is like developing new and refined "software."

Both scenarios seem to go hand in hand, correct? Does neuroplasticity mean that what you call "hardware" and "software" are two sides of the same coin and they influence each other?

Correct. So these days we do not make a sharp distinction, and are conducting more neuroimaging studies to better understand the relationship between both.

BUILDING THE COGNITIVE RESERVE

If the goal is to build that cognitive reserve of neurons, synapses, and skills, how can we do that? What defines mentally stimulating activities or good brain exercise?

In summary, we could say that "brain stimulation" consists of engaging in activities. In our research almost all activities are seen to contribute to building the reserve. Some have challenging levels of cognitive complexity, and some have interpersonal or physical demands. In animal studies, exposure to an enriched environment or increased physical activity results in increased neurogenesis (the creation of new neurons). You can get that stimulation through education and/or your occupation. There is clear research showing how those two elements reduce the risk.

What is very exciting is that, no matter one's age, education and occupation, our level of participation in leisure activities has a significant and cumulative effect. A key message here is that different activities have independent, synergistic effects. This means that the more things you do and the earlier you start, the better. But you are never stuck. It is better to start late than never.

Can you give us some examples of leisure activities that seem to have the most positive effects?

For our 2001 study we evaluated the effect of thirteen activities, combining intellectual, physical, and social elements. Some of the activities with the most effect were reading, visiting friends or relatives, going to movies or restaurants, and walking for pleasure or going on an excursion. As you can see, there are a variety of options.

We saw that the group with a high level of leisure activities presented thirty-eight percent less risk (controlling for other factors) of developing Alzheimer's symptoms. And that, for each additional type of activity, the risk got reduced by eight percent.

There is also an additional element that we are starting to see more clearly. Physical exercise, by itself, also has a very beneficial impact on cognition. Only a few months ago researchers were able to show for the first time how physical activity promotes neurogenesis in the human brain.

So, we need both mental and physical exercise. The not-so-good news is that, as of today, there is no clear recipe for success. More research is needed before we can prepare a systematic set of interventions that can help maximize our protection.

We often hear about the importance of good nutrition, physical exercise, stress management and mental exercise that present novelty, variety and challenge. What do you think of the relatively recent appearance of so many computer-based cognitive training programs, some more science-based than others?

The elements you mention make sense. The problem is that, at least from the point of view of Alzheimer's, we cannot be much more specific. We do not know if learning a new language is more beneficial than learning a new musical instrument or using a computer-based program.

A few of the cognitive training computer programs we have seen, like the one you discussed with Professor Daniel Gopher to train the mental abilities of pilots, seem to have clear effects on cognition, generalizing beyond the training itself. But, for the most part, it is too early to tell the long-term effects. We need better designed clinical trials with clear controls. Right now, the most we can say is that those who lead mentally stimulating lives, through education, occupation and leisure activities seem to have the least risk of developing Alzheimer's disease.

Interview with Dr. Elizabeth Zelinski – Healthy aging and cognitive enhancement.

BACKGROUND:

Dr. Elizabeth Zelinski of the Southern California Andrus Gerontology Center led the IMPACT (Improvement in Memory with Plasticity-based Adaptive Cognitive Training) study.

The IMPACT study, which is by far the largest high-quality study of its kind, was prospective, randomized, controlled, and used a double blind trial. 524 healthy adults sixty-five or older were divided into two groups. One received an hour a day of brain training for eight to ten weeks, and the other spent the same amount of time watching educational DVDs. Funded by Posit Science corporation, the study was performed in multiple locations, including the Mayo Clinic, USCF, and San Francisco Veteran Affairs Medical Center.

HIGHLIGHTS:

- The aging brain has a harder time dealing with novelty, but gets better at dealing with the familiar.

- There is not one general intelligence but many different cognitive abilities. This is why different programs need to be designed to train and improve each of them.

HOW COGNITIVE ABILITIES EVOLVE AS WE AGE

What insights did you gain from your Long Beach Longitudinal Study into how human cognitive abilities typically evolve as we age?

The first concept to understand is that different cognitive skills evolve over our lifespan in different ways. Some that rely on experience, such as vocabulary, actually improve as we age. Some tend to decline gradually, starting in our late twenties. This happens, for example, with processing speed (how long it takes us to process and respond to information), memory, and reasoning. We could summarize this phenomenon by saying that as we age we get better at dealing with the familiar, but worse at dealing with the new. We can always learn, but at a slower pace.

Is there a specific tipping or inflection point in this trend, any age when the rate of decline is more pronounced?

We do not have a clear answer to that. It depends a lot on the individual. In general it is a gradual, cumulative process, so that by age seventy we statistically see clear age declines. Which, for example, is a strong factor determining why older adults struggle to adapt to new technologies, but why trying to learn them provides needed mental stimulation. We know that genes only account for a portion of this decline. Much of it depends on our environment, lifestyle and actions.

Can you summarize what a healthy individual can do to slow down this process of decline, and help stay healthy and productive as long as possible?

One general recommendation is to do everything we can to prevent or delay disease processes, such as diabetes or high-blood pressure, that have a negative effect on our brains. For example, it is a tragedy in our society that we usually reduce our levels of physical exercise drastically after we leave school.

IMPACTS OF PHYSICAL VS. MENTAL EXERCISE

What are the relative virtues of physical vs. mental exercise?

This question leads to my second recommendation. Aerobic exercise has been shown to be a great contributor to overall cognitive health.

But it has not shown any significant effect on improved memory. This is an important point to remember: there have been dozens of studies on the impact of physical exercise on cognition and they have found many impacts, but none in the area of memory. In contrast, directed cognitive training, or mental exercise, has been shown to improve specific cognitive abilities, including memory.

Now, there is no magic bullet. Both physical and mental exercise are important components. And I would add a third element: it is also important to maintain emotional connections. Not only with ourselves, to have self- confidence and self-esteem, but also with our family our friends.

IMPACT STUDY

What results of the IMPACT study surprised you the most?

Probably the most surprising outcome was a clear transfer of the training, which is critical so that the cognitive improvements have an impact on everyday life. The program we used, Brain Fitness 2.0, trains auditory processing. The people in the experimental group improved very significantly, which was not that surprising. What was very surprising was that there was also a clear benefit in auditory memory, which was not directly trained. In other words, we found that after using the program, people who were seventy-five years old performed auditory memory tasks as well as average sixty-five year olds, so we can say they reversed ten years of aging for that cognitive ability.

Another area where people in the experimental group showed significant improvement was in self-reported perception of their abilities in a variety of daily life tasks, such as remembering names and phone numbers, where they had left their keys, as well as communication abilities and feelings of self-confidence.

ENVISIONING A FUTURE WITH BRAIN GYMS

Those results, even if initial, are impressive and have very significant implications. Let us now speculate a bit about the future. We have said that different cognitive abilities evolve in different ways, and we have talked about just a few of them. We have discussed how physical exercise can be useful. And how directed cognitive training may help improve specific cognitive skills, like the Brain Fitness 2.0 program developed by Dr. Michael Merzenich. Other examples include working memory training, shown by Dr. Torkel Klingberg, and attentional control, by Dr. Daniel Gopher. In the future, will we have access to better assessments and tools to identify and train the cognitive abilities we need to work on the most, in the same way that we can go to a gym today and find the combination of machines that provide the most effective personalized workout?

The physical fitness analogy is a good one, in that cognitive enhancement requires engagement in a variety of activities. Those activities must be novel, adaptive and challenging. This is why computer-based programs can be helpful. Even at a more basic level, what matters is being engaged with life, continually exposed to stimulating activities, always trying to get out of our comfort zones, and doing our best at whatever we are doing.

A typical misconception about the brain is that there is only one general intelligence to care about. In reality, we have many different cognitive abilities, such as attention, memory, language, reasoning, and more, so it makes sense to have different programs designed to train and improve each of them. Before embarking on this study I was skeptical about what we would find. Now I believe that cognitive training is a very promising area that deserves more scientific and policy attention.

What is one recent finding or reflection, from your own work or others', that you'd like more people of all ages to know about as they try to maintain/enhance their own brain fitness?

It is critically important to find brain fitness activities that people will be willing to commit to, and to make those activities part of their lifestyle. It may be best to combine different types of activities (e.g. aerobic exercise, computer games, extended cognitive practice) to optimize benefit since, as we discussed in our recent meta-analysis, it is the practice over time that brings important benefits.

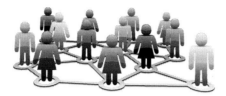

CHAPTER 6

OH, THE PEOPLE YOU'LL MEET!

We have seen the potential benefits of general mental exercise. You may have noticed that several of the scientists interviewed also mentioned the benefits of social stimulation. Growing evidence strongly suggests that social engagement contributes to optimizing brain health. But are all types of social engagement equal? What matters most – quantity or quality?

BENEFITS OF SOCIAL ENGAGEMENT

Studies, often focused on at-risk populations, have found that social isolation is detrimental for overall health. Isolated people see their risks of all-cause mortality increase two to four times compared to those with social contact with either friends and family or a general community. In terms of brain health in particular, the recent NIH extensive meta-analysis confirms that higher social engagement in mid- to late life is associated with higher cognitive functioning and reduced risk of cognitive decline. Evidence associating low social engagement in mid- to late life with increased risk of Alzheimer's disease is even stronger.

The effect of social engagement can be observed directly in the brain. A 2011 study focused on the amygdala, a structure in the limbic system that plays a major role in our emotional responses. The researchers reasoned that the amygdala would be a likely candidate to be modified (via neuroplastic changes) by the level of social engagement one has. They measured the size of the amydgala of 60 adults and assessed the size and complexity of their social networks (i.e., how many people they were in regular contact with and the number of different groups these contacts could be divided into). Results showed that the size of the amygdala was not related to the amount of social support the participants felt they had. However, the larger and the more complex a person's social network actually was, the bigger their amygdala. The question then becomes: do people with bigger amygdala tend to make more friends or is it making more friends that triggers growth in the amygdala? This question is still an open one, as non-correlational, causal evidence is needed to answer it.

Such evidence is just starting to become available. In 2008, Oscar Ybarra and his colleagues at the University of Michigan randomly assigned participants (aged 18-21) to three groups: 1) a social group, in which the participants engaged in a discussion of a social issue for 10 minutes, 2) an intellectual activities group, in which the participants solved stimulating tasks (crossword puzzles and the like) for 10 minutes, and 3) a control group, in which the participants watched a 10-minute clip of the television show Seinfeld. After they participated in the discussion, watched the clip, or solved the puzzles, the cognitive functioning of all the participants was assessed using a speed of processing task and a working memory (WM) task. Results showed that people in the intellectual activities group did better in the WM task than people who merely watched a video. The same cognitive boost was observed in the social interaction group, suggesting that WM was exercised during the discussion and benefited from that stimulation. And the study suggested, once more, that the average TV watcher would benefit from watching less TV and spending some of that "saved" time on cognitively stimulating activities.

WHY WOULD SOCIAL ENGAGEMENT BOOST BRAIN FUNCTIONS?

As Oscar Ybarra (whose interview you can find at the end of this chapter) points out, "participating in a discussion involves using social cognitive processes, such as inferring what people are thinking, taking someone else's perspective, memorizing and updating information, and inhibiting inappropriate emotions and behaviors." Thus social interactions provide "embedded" brain exercise, stimulating executive functions and contributing to both short-term performance boosts and the buildup of cognitive reserve.

Of course not all social interactions are equal, and some require more cognitive engagement than others and are thus probably more beneficial in terms of brain fitness – think about the same guidelines of novelty, variety, and challenge discussed in the previous chapter. You can expect to accrue more benefits within groups that have a purpose (such as a book club or a spiritual group) compared to casual social interactions (such as having a drink with a friend to relax after work). In a 2011 study, Ybarra showed that a cooperative interaction or a basic get-to-know-you interaction are the kinds of interaction that trigger a short-term cognitive boost.

Laura Fratiglioni and her colleagues have suggested that the relationship between social stimulation and decreased risks of dementia can also be explained by the vascular and stress hypotheses. The vascular hypothesis links social engagement to beneficial effects on cardiovascular diseases and stroke. Since vascular diseases are involved in the triggering and progression of dementia, it is likely that a factor reducing these risks would also reduce the emergence of dementia.

As outlined in Chapter 7, stress is associated with hippocampal atrophy, cognitive decline, and dementia. The stress hypothesis states that individuals with more social contacts have more opportunities to engage with other people and thus more opportunities to feel that they are well integrated and socially competent. This may increase their self-esteem and mood and lower their stress levels, which in turn would contribute to lowering their risks of cognitive decline and dementia. In this context, it seems that any kind of social relationship can be beneficial, regardless of whether or not it involves a high level of intellectual stimulation, as long as it involves a friendly encounter.

WHAT MATTERS IN A SOCIAL NETWORK?

You can have numerous friends, a few close ones, or both. At the same time, you can be surrounded by many people but still not feel supported socially. Do we know what matters the most in terms of brain health: social network size, quality of relationship, or perhaps subjective estimate of social support? The evidence so far does not offer conclusive results and is too limited for very precise guidelines.

A 2009 study looked at the social habits and cognitive functioning of 838 healthy individuals, 80 years old on average. Social engagement was assessed with measures of social activity frequency, size of social networks, and perceived social support. To measure frequency of social activity, participants were asked to rate how often during the past year they engaged in six types of activities that involve social interaction: 1) going to restaurants, sporting events, or playing bingo; 2) going on day or overnight trips; 3) doing volunteer work; 4) visiting relatives or friends; 5) participating in groups; 6) attending religious services. To measure the size of their social networks, participants were asked about the number of children, family, and friends they had and how often they had seen them in the past year. Social support was assessed with a few items from a standardized scale specifically designed for this purpose. Cognitive functioning of the participants was assessed with a battery of 19 tests measuring long-term memory, working memory, processing speed, and visuospatial ability.

The researchers then used statistical analysis to try to understand how each of the 3 measures of social engagement was related to the participants' level of cognitive functioning. They found that more frequent participation in social activities and a higher level of perceived social support were associated with higher cognitive functioning, while interestingly enough, social network size was not related. This may suggest that high-quality, satisfying relationships may matter more than how many relationships one has.

However, other studies have found an association between the size of one's social support group and cognitive functioning, showing both in healthy older adults and in individuals with dementia that a larger social network size is associated with better cognitive function.

EXPANDING SOCIAL LIFE

In other words, we need to focus on the basics: more social engagement is better than less, especially interactions that naturally involve novelty, variety, and challenge in addition to a degree of social support. There are many different ways to increase your social engagement. These will depend on your age, goals, and current level of social connection and support. Although no solution is perfect for everybody, here are a few suggestions.

Volunteering

One way to meet new people and stay socially engaged is through volunteer work (at a library, hospital, school, etc.). Several studies show that volunteering is greatly beneficial: it lowers mortality and depression rates, and slows down rates of decline in health and function.

A recently created community-based program called Experience Corps highlights the benefits of volunteering. In this program, seniors partner with schools to help children improve academically and behaviorally. Participants volunteer 15 hours per week. They get social support through team training and service. They also get cognitive stimulation, especially for executive functions, as they switch between mentoring academic activities, assisting in the school library, and helping with conflict resolution. Michelle Carlson and her colleagues at the Johns Hopkins Bloomberg School of Public Health conducted a 6-month brain imaging study to evaluate the effects of Experience Corps. They found that participants in the program showed improved executive functions compared to controls, as well as increased activity in the part of the brain that supports these functions (the prefrontal cortex).

Social groups

Another way to boost social engagement is to belong to a group, such as a book club or a religious group. Since belonging to a group usually involves doing something with its members, benefits can vary depending on the activity performed with the group.

In 2007, Hui-Chuan Hsu from Asia University studied data from an elderly population in Taiwan and found that participating in a religious group reduced the risk of mortality for women and participating in a political group reduced the risk of cognitive dysfunction in men. Setting aside the gender difference, which may be specific to this population, these results suggest that different types of social groups may have different effects. Hsu reasons that the effect of participating in a political group may be partly caused by the intellectual stimulation one gets while discussing political issues. In contrast, the effect of belonging to a religious group may be partly caused by an increase in well-being.

In sum, any kind of social group will combine the benefit of social engagement with those triggered by the activity performed by the group. A dance club or a walking book club will combine benefits from social and physical activity, while a bridge club will combine intellectual and social engagement.

Someone who is not very socially oriented may be hesitant to participate in new activities involving unfamiliar people. This person may need a little help to start. But the good news is that openness to new experiences does not seem to be a fixed personality trait. A study recently showed that stimulating cognitive skills may enhance openness in older adults. Half of the 183 participants were trained for 16 weeks. They were provided with increasingly difficult pattern-recognition and problem-solving tasks in a class-based setting and with puzzles that they could perform at home. Compared to non-trained participants, they showed better inductive reasoning scores at the end of the study, showing that the cognitive training was effective. The training group also experienced significant increases in openness.

This is an important result for two reasons. First, openness is known to decrease with age so it is good to know that such a trend can be reversed. Second, it gives hope that once someone starts a stimulating activity in a social context, the benefits gained will trigger both adherence to the activity and maybe the wish to start new ones.

WHAT ABOUT SOCIAL MEDIA?

More and more adults have a Facebook page for friends, a LinkedIn account for business, or at least send emails or texts to stay in touch with their social network. This recent trend raises many questions: how valuable are these electronic social interactions? Do they have the same beneficial effects on the brain as face-to-face interactions? Does one get more friends by using social media? The effect of Internet use on social relationships is still a matter of intense debate and controversy.

Digital relationships are different from face-to-face ones in many aspects. Since we cannot see the person (except when using a video-chat program such as Skype), we cannot read her or his facial expressions and body language, opening the door to potential misinterpretations about the emotions and intentions of the person we are talking too. Trust is thus much more of an issue in digital relationships than in face-to-face ones. This may explain why people generally find interactions with their close friends more satisfying when they happen face-to-face than via other media such as phone, texting, and social networking sites. There is something critical in the ability to see another person speak and react to what we say.

Does Facebook actually bring us more friends? Let's start by looking at how many friends people have in general. A 1992 study found a correlation between typical social group size and cortical volume in a wide range of primates and human communities. This suggests that the number of individuals with whom it is possible to maintain stable relationships (i.e., number of friends) is constrained by our cortical processing capacity. In humans the size of the brain's cortex seems to limit social network size to about 150 individuals. This number is now known as Dunbar's number. Can social media, and especially social networking sites, increase this number?

Although some people have thousands of "virtual friends" on Facebook, it turns out that the typical number is around 120, which corresponds to Dunbar's number – that is, the number of friends people typically have in real life. This was confirmed for Twitter too. Of course, even in real life it is possible to know more than 150 people. Some people have hundreds of acquaintances (in addition to close friends) and are able to recognize thousands of people. On Facebook too some people have a thousand or more "friends." However these people are unlikely to be actual friends, in the sense that they are probably not people who would help out in a difficult situation.

Is social networking destroying our "real" friendships? Evidence is mixed so far, but good news is that the size of one's online social network doesn't seem to negatively affect one's offline network.

Maybe one of the best aspects of social network sites is that they allow us to keep in contact with friends we can no longer see, which prevents the friendships from fading away. It seems valuable and stimulating to have friends in different geographical locations, especially these days when we tend to travel and move more often than ever before.

CHAPTER HIGHLIGHTS

- A social interaction can be a complex and cognitively demanding activity involving executive functions, which makes exposure to stimulating social environments a priority for optimizing brain functioning.

- Social engagement benefits the brain by contributing to building cognitive/brain reserve and lowering stress levels.

- Online social networks do not seem to increase (or decrease) the number of friendships we can maintain, possibly because of natural constraints imposed by the size of our cortex.

INTERVIEWS

- Dr. Oscar Ybarra – Some social interactions, but not all, can boost cognition.

Interview with Dr. Oscar Ybarra –
Some social interactions, but not all, can boost cognition.

BACKGROUND

Dr. Oscar Ybarra is Professor of Psychology at the University of Michigan. He is the director of the Adaptive Social Cognition Lab in which social regulation skills and cognitive capital and their interplay are studied. He is among the few researchers so far who have provided causal evidence that engaging in a social interaction can have a positive short-term effect on cognitive performance.

HIGHLIGHTS:

- A social interaction that creates a cognitive boost is one in which the person is engaged and motivated, that is, uses executive functions (by engaging in perspective taking, mind reading, monitoring, and inhibition skills).

- Casual chats and competitive interactions do not usually trigger cognitive benefits.

Your research revolves around social intelligence. Can you define what it is?

Social intelligence is the ability to understand one's social surroundings, problem solve and manage relationships, while balancing personal needs with the needs of others.

SOCIAL INTERACTIONS:
SOME ARE GOOD AND SOME ARE BAD

The paper you published in 2008 "Mental exercise through simple socializing" is one of the few studies showing a causal relation between social interaction and cognitive enhancement. Can you briefly summarize the study and its findings?

The study had three conditions. One group of participants watched TV for 10 minutes. This was the control group, which had a social component since participants were watching people interact on the screen.

Another group performed brain exercises (such as crosswords, and mental rotation task) for 10 minutes, and another one had a 10min discussion on a specific topic. Working memory performance (a main element of executive functions) was tested afterwards. Participating in the discussion resulted in a performance boost (compared to the control condition) that was as high as the boost resulting from the brain exercises.

The performance boost can be explained by the fact that participating in a discussion involves using social cognitive processes, such as inferring what people are thinking, taking someone else's perspective, memorizing and updating information, and inhibiting inappropriate emotions and behaviors. Many of these abilities rely on executive functions, and when executive functions are engaged in this manner during social interaction, they become resources that are later applicable to tasks such as tests of working memory and cognitive control.

Social interactions have been found to have negative effects on cognition and be cognitively depleting. Can you explain these findings?

Some research has shown that challenging or "high-maintenance" interactions can result in a reduction in cognitive functioning. These interactions usually involve self-presentation concerns that last during the whole interaction (for instance about appearing unintelligent) as well as effortful attempts to self-regulate. All this could result in the temporary depletion of cognitive resources, especially executive functions. However in most interaction studies that have found cognitive depletion, there was no control group to use as a comparison. So it is possible that what looks like a negative effect may in fact merely be an absence of a boost from social interaction.

WHAT IN THE INTERACTION CREATES
A COGNITIVE BOOST?

What are the required ingredients in a social interaction that will trigger a cognitive boost?

One has to be engaged and motivated, that is try to understand the other person, try to read her mind, take her perspective, monitor the content of the conversation as well as ones behavior. A cooperative interaction or a basic get-to-know-you interaction usually combine all these ingredients and trigger a cognitive boost. By contrast, as we showed in our 2011 paper, interactions involving a competitive goal do not exercise executive functions as much, probably because they trigger withdrawal from the interaction and self-protection. As a consequence they do not result in a cognitive boost.

So a visit to a family member or friend is not likely to be a cognitively boosting interaction?

Not if it is a routine visit or involves a relationship you take for granted. It may be a pleasant interaction but will probably not create a boost. Again this is all about being engaged and motivated and really trying to take perspective and understand where the other person is coming from. A casual chat will not do the trick.

SOCIAL INTELLIGENCE
AND COMPUTERIZED TRAINING

Could the knowledge that social interactions benefit cognition be integrated in computerized programs that aim at boosting targeted functions such as working memory?

People are social and need to connect with others. So one could introduce social elements in the computer programs to make them more engaging. The social element may boost the motivation to use the program over time as well.

Some people do not engage in many social interactions either because they are shy or because they lack social competence. What solutions can you think of to help them?

Experimentally one could isolate certain social skills and test whether these capacities can be trained. This may help people or children develop basic skills, for example, even just learning to wait and take turns and listen during interaction. The training would be helpful in the social domain but also more generally since it should involve the exercising of executive functions. For instance, Adele Diamond and colleagues have shown that social behaviors such as active listening, taking turns and checking each other's progress on tasks can result in better performance on executive function tasks.

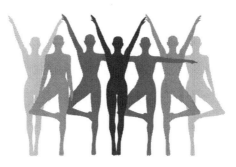

CHAPTER 7

MANAGE STRESS, BUILD RESILIENCE

The society we live in is increasingly fast-paced and complex. The amount of knowledge we are supposed to acquire and retain throughout life is enormous. The lifelong demands on any person have changed more rapidly in the last thousand years than our genes and brains have, putting to the test our ability to regulate stress and emotions. Which begs the question: what is the impact of stress on the brain? How does stress affect our functioning now and in the future? How can we learn to manage stress and build resilience?

POSITIVE AND NEGATIVE STRESS

Cognition and emotion are tightly intertwined, both structurally (as discussed in Chapter 1, they occur in strongly interconnected and overlapping parts of the brain) and functionally (for example, high levels of anxiety can reduce working memory capacity). A good example is the ability of emotions to change the formation and recollection of an event: in general, emotional events are remembered much better than non-emotional ones, and for a much longer period of time.

Stress is a common emotion (and not just for humans). It is triggered by an experience or situation in which the demands on an organism exceed its natural capacity to regulate itself. Organisms generally work hard to maintain equilibrium, or "homeostasis." Stimuli coming from the environment or from the organism itself may disturb this equilibrium. Stress is often defined as both the factor that causes the organism to move away from equilibrium and the process by which the organism tries to return to equilibrium. The attempt to get back to equilibrium often consumes energy and resources, such as in the fight-or-flight response that occurs when we are faced with an external source of danger.

Stress is not always bad – there is such thing as "positive" stress. Such stress is often experienced as butterflies in the stomach or sweaty palms before a big athletic game, artistic performance or speech, or at work before an important presentation, phone call, or meeting. This "positive" stress may increase alertness and boost performance. The physiological manifestations are present for a short period of time in our body and then get used up as the goal is accomplished. Once the goal is accomplished, there is typically time to rest and recover while basking in the glow of a successful performance.

Some stress can be good, but as we'll see, too much stress is not. The key for good functioning is to be able to understand and manage stress, and to build resilience over time.

THE BRAIN STRESS RESPONSE

Let's take a look inside the brain to understand what happens when we are stressed. In Chapter 1, we discussed various brain structures. The neocortex is where higher-level thought processes occur. The limbic system is composed of several structures, including the amygdala, the hippocampus, and the hypothalamus, that work together to manage (in conjunction with the neocortex) emotions, motivation, the regulation of memories, breathing and heart rate, the production of hormones, sexual arousal, and circadian rhythms. As you have probably already guessed, the limbic system plays a prominent role in the so-called stress response. In fact, when we are stressed, the limbic system sends the alarm signal and the neocortex (in particular the prefrontal cortex) makes sense of the alarm.

The first thing to happen when a person experiences physical or mental stress is the release of a signal by the hypothalamus that activates the sympathetic nervous system (SNS), which manages the fight-or-flight response. The SNS is a part of the peripheral nervous system, which consists of the spinal cord and all the nerves that are in the body outside the brain. SNS functions range from constricting blood vessels (which increases blood pressure), activating sweat glands, and dilating pupils, to increasing heart rate and its force of contraction.

The SNS manages all that by mediating the increase in production of a stress hormone called adrenaline (or epinephrine) which, in combination with norepinephrine, speeds up the heart rate and increases metabolism and blood pressure. The SNS also triggers the increased release of another hormone called cortisol, which helps enhance the memory, immune system, and anti-inflammatory responses, as well as lower sensitivity to pain. In other words, increased activity in the SNS will get you ready for immediate survival challenges.

When the stress is overcome, the hypothalamus normally signals to lower the release of the stress hormones. The parasympathetic nervous system (PNS) is then engaged to get the body back to normal. The PNS deals with the "rest-and-digest" activities that occur when the body is at rest (i.e., salivation, urination, sexual arousal, and digestion). As you can see, the SNS and PNS naturally work together to keep us in equilibrium.

In his excellent book, *Why Zebras Don't Have Ulcers*, Robert Sapolsky points out that humans are unique in that we are among the few animals that can get stressed from their own thoughts. When we are stressed for any reason we have the same kind of stress reaction that, for example, a zebra would when it tries to escape from the clutches of a lion. However, in trying to save its life by running away, the zebra essentially uses up its stress hormones to fuel its escape. Humans, on the other hand, usually just keep muddling along and let the stress build up over long periods of time.

In contrast with the (potentially) beneficial effects of short bursts of stress, high and sustained levels of stress – chronic stress – can have a number of negative consequences. The more stress, the more cortisol in the blood. Too much cortisol can lead to problems such as blood sugar imbalances, high blood pressure, loss of muscle tissue and bone density, and lower immunity and inflammatory responses. It can also cause damage to the brain and block the formation of new connections in the hippocampus, the key actor in encoding new memories in the brain. For instance, Sonia Lupien and her colleagues at McGill University showed that in older adults, long-term exposure to high levels of cortisol is associated with both memory impairments and a 14% smaller hippocampal volume.

Chronic stress hampers our ability to both make changes to reduce the stress and to even be creative enough to think of possible changes we could make. Overall, stress limits mental flexibility and the ability to see alternative solutions. As such, it can prevent us from adapting to, and succeeding in, new circumstances. General Adaptation Syndrome (GAS) describes the effects of the long-term kind of stress that does not go away and paralyzes someone into inaction. This state is popularly called burnout. People experiencing this type of stress often lose motivation and drive and feel mentally exhausted. They are emotionally flat and may become cynical and non-responsive to others.

In sum, we possess the basic equipment to handle stress. But we need to learn how to use that equipment to prevent or mitigate the problems that arise when we are confronted with too much stress.

STRESS AND DEPRESSION

Stress and depression are separate states, but they are closer than commonly thought.

First, chronic stress is associated with a reduction of certain neurotransmitters in the brain, such as serotonin and dopamine, which have been linked to depression. These chemicals normally help regulate sleep, appetite, energy, sex drive and emotions. Second, people suffering from major depression show increased levels of cortisol. High levels of stress are associated with too much cortisol, and research suggests that in some people this may lead to depression. Finally, people who are heavily stressed tend to neglect healthy lifestyle behaviors such as regular exercise while favoring unhealthy behaviors such as smoking and drinking more than usual in order to get some relief, which may increase the risk of depression.

According to the recent NIH extensive meta-analysis, depression is associated with both higher risks of cognitive decline and higher risks of developing Alzheimer's disease. Depression is also known to have an immediate impact on one's cognitive functions, such as lower motivation and decreased attention and memory. Managing stress, building resilience, and preventing depression are therefore important factors to be considered in the context of optimizing brain health and performance.

LIFESTYLE SOLUTIONS AGAINST STRESS

As highlighted above, following a prolonged exposure to high stress levels, it can be difficult to really return to homeostasis, which can damage the brain and hamper good cognitive functioning. As part of a brain-healthy lifestyle it is thus essential to manage stress efficiently and effectively. What can you do when you realize that you are stressed?

Here are a few research-based lifestyle solutions that can be used against stress:

Exercise: Over time, chronic stress contributes to neuronal death and slows down neurogenesis. In contrast, studies show that aerobic physical exercise helps build up new neurons and connections (as discussed in Chapter 3). Exercise is thus a great tool to counteract the effects of stress on the brain. This has been shown in a study looking at middle-age and older adults. The 2012 study reported that people who did not exercise much exhibited greater stress-related atrophy of the hippocampus compared to people who exercised more.

Regular exercise also promotes good sleep, which is usually disturbed by stress. In addition, exercise can reduce the experience of stress and depression, as well as increase self-confidence, by boosting the production of endorphins, the "feel-good" neurotransmitters. As their name indicates (endo- is short for endogenous, that is, coming from inside and –orphin is short for morphine), endorphins have an analgesic effect and produce a feeling of well-being. They are produced during exercise as well as during excitement, pain, expressions of love, and orgasm.

Relaxation: Relaxation, whether through meditation (see below), tai chi, yoga, or a walk on the beach, lowers blood pressure, slows respiration and metabolism, and releases muscle tension. As such it is a good tool to counteract the negative effects of stress. An intriguing 2008 study by University of Michigan researchers Marc Berman, John Jonides, and Stephen Kaplan compared the restorative effects on cognitive function of walking in either a natural or an urban environment. The cognitive function they focused on was voluntary attention. Participants in the study first performed a 35-minute task that fatigued their attention. Then they walked for 50 minutes either in a city or in a large park. Upon their return, participants who took a walk in the park showed much better performance on a test of voluntary attention than those who took a walk in the city. Interestingly, in a second study, the same restorative effect of nature was observed after people spent ten minutes merely looking at 50 pictures of nature (rather than pictures of a city). The researchers explained their results by the fact that unlike a natural environment, urban environments contain many attention grabbing stimuli (e.g., a shiny, fast-moving car) that also require directed attention (e.g., to avoid being hit by that car). As a consequence, nature allows voluntary attention abilities to replenish much more than an urban environment does.

Socialization: Cultivating social networks of friends, family, and even pets, can help foster trust, support, and relaxation. There is ample evidence that satisfying social relationships are crucial for both mental and physical health. Specifically, we know that loneliness increases risks of cardiovascular diseases and levels of stress and decreases quality of sleep. It has been linked with depression too. Loneliness is more strongly associated with how many close relationships one has than with mere contact with one's social network members. This suggests that maintaining good relationships with a few close friends may be key to managing stress and staying healthy.

Empowerment: What does empowerment mean exactly? It means feeling in control over important aspects of our own lives – including brain health. Correlation studies suggest an association between psychological empowerment and stress resiliency. Finding ways to empower oneself can thus be a defense against chronic stress.

Humor and laughter: Intuitively, we can sense that a good laugh seems to be a useful aid for fighting off stress, and indeed research suggests that it can help. For instance, in 2002 Mary Bennett and her colleagues reported that viewing a humorous video (as opposed to viewing a tourism video) decreased self-reported stress in a group of healthy adult women. In 2004, a neuroimaging study showed that self-generated happiness or sadness activated the same parts of the brain as real emotions. In addition, imagined laughter was successful at reducing self-reported sadness and imagined crying at reducing self-reported happiness. Another small study in 1989 showed that viewing a 60-min. comedy video decreased participant's levels of cortisol and epinephrine, which suggests that laughter could help counteract the hormonal effects of stress. Globally the evidence supporting the direct benefits of laughter is not entirely conclusive as of yet, but all studies show positive effects, especially when laughter is used in therapeutic contexts.

Positive Thinking: Thinking positively about stressors can help moderate stress. In 2010, for example, Jeremy Jamieson and colleagues at Harvard University coached students into believing that feeling nervous and/or excited before an exam could in fact improve performance. In other words they coached them into having positive thoughts and thereby reappraising their stress. The students received this coaching before taking practice graduate-school entrance exams in the lab. Compared with students who were not coached, these students got higher scores both during the practice test and on the actual exam 3 months later.

Thinking about positive events in general may also help enhance your mood and happiness and lower your levels of stress. Dr. Emmons, whose interview you can find at the end of this chapter, has shown that keeping a "gratitude journal" where you regularly write something you are grateful for significantly increases self-reported levels of happiness and wellbeing.

MEDITATION: A CAPACITY-BUILDING TECHNIQUE TO MANAGE STRESS AND BUILD RESILIENCE

The lifestyle solutions described above constitute useful tools to help manage stress and build emotional resilience. Additionally, effective emotional regulation depends on being able to flexibly adjust our physiological responses to a changing environment, and there are efficient techniques for learning how to directly use our basic equipment or physiological system to build up the capacity for dealing with stress over time. While chapter 8 will focus extensively on how to "cross-train" the brain, for many of us facing stressful and complex realities, the cross-training should probably start here, with training the brain to deal more efficiently with stress and emotions. One way to do so by building up a capacity for monitoring or influencing these responses is through meditation.

There are many ways to meditate. The ultimate goal is to go beyond one's automatic thinking to get into a "deeper" or more grounded state. This can be achieved by:

- trying to think about nothing *(basic meditation)*

- focusing on a particular object, either outside of oneself (such as a sound or candle flame, or a mantra) or inside (such as one's breathing) *(focused meditation)*

- engaging in a repetitive activity such as yoga or walking *(activity-oriented meditation)* or singing *(Kirtan Kriya meditation)*

- becoming more fully aware, more "mindful" of the present moment, rather than thinking about the past or the future *(mindfulness meditation)*

- engaging in a spiritual practice such as prayer *(spiritual meditation)*

Meditation helps to exercise and build up 1) the control of attention and 2) the control of emotional arousal. We will now discuss the emotional control benefit (see Chapter 8 for a more detailed discussion of meditation as a technique to train attentional control).

A common theme across meditation techniques is the focus on deep and slow breathing. Controlling one's breathing may help reduce physical symptoms of stress such as high arousal and reactivity and increased heart rate. As described earlier, our heart rate variability (HRV) is managed by the actions of both the sympathetic nervous system (SNS) and the parasympathetic nervous system (PNS). Faster heart rates are due to increased SNS activity while slower heart rates can be attributed to increased PNS activity.

The actions of the SNS and PNS are automatic. How can you consciously manage involuntary actions? Research shows that this not only is it possible, but it can be accomplished by learning something as relatively simple as how to regulate your breathing. Breathing air into the lungs temporarily gates off the parasympathetic influence on heart rate, producing a heart rate increase. Breathing air out of the lungs reinstates parasympathetic influence on heart rate, resulting in a heart rate decrease. By changing one's breathing, it is thus possible to increase the PNS influence on the heart, helping the body to return to equilibrium faster (sometimes also referred to as "coherence").

Evidence that meditative techniques can help manage stress is clear. Mindfulness Based Stress Reduction (MBSR) programs have been used in several studies with healthy but stressed participants. These 8 week programs use mindfulness meditation and yoga to teach participants to react non-judgmentally to stressful events by focusing on their breathing or their body or by walking. The hypothesis is that mastering these skills enhances the efficiency of top-down control processes that regulate emotional responses, which in turn may lead to a reduction in stress responses. Several studies have shown that such programs successfully reduce stress. For instance, a small 2008 randomized study involving 60 middle-aged individuals showed that a MBSR intervention resulted in reduced levels of perceived stress, and in increased levels of perceived quality of life and positive affect.

Recent evidence shows that a MBSR program can lead to changes in one of the brain structures that deals with emotions: the amygdala.

In this study, the brains of 26 healthy but stressed individuals were scanned before and after a MBRS intervention. Results showed that reported stress was lower after the intervention and that this reduction in stress correlated with decreases in the density of an area of the amygdala.

In the clinical world, one of the most studied techniques to alleviate symptoms of depression, stress, and unhappiness is mindfulness-based cognitive therapy (MBCT or MBT). This therapy combines features of cognitive therapy and mindfulness meditation. The goal is to learn how to pay attention without judgment, and to recognize feelings that are ineffective and mentally destructive so that one can respond rationally to these feelings instead of reacting to them impulsively. MBCT usually consists of eight weekly two-hour classes with assignments to be completed at home.

A recent meta-analysis assessed the role of MBT as reported in 39 studies. All the studies in the analysis included adult participants between 18 and 65 years-old who had a psychological disorder (anxiety-related or depression) or a medical disorder (e.g., cancer or chronic pain). MBT was successful at improving anxiety and depression in patients with anxiety disorders and depression. It also improved symptoms of anxiety and depression when these symptoms were associated with medical disorders. The beneficial impact of MBT was observed across a relatively wide range of symptom severity and was maintained on average for 12 weeks after the therapy. Such results support the use of MBT for anxiety and depression in clinical populations.

Other types of meditation have also been shown to have a positive impact on stress and cognition. You can read some of D. Newberg's findings below, based on his research on Kirtan Kriya meditation. Another recent review article suggested that transcendental meditation (TM) helps reduce risk of cardiovascular disease because, among other things, it helps decrease psychological stress and blood pressure.

CHAPTER HIGHLIGHTS

- Some stress is good (it can increase alertness), some is bad (high and sustained levels of stress can alter several physical functions and cause the death of brain cells). The key for good mental functioning is to regulate your stress.

- Stress management can be achieved by using lifestyle solutions (such as positive thinking and physical exercise) and targeted, capacity-building techniques and products (such as meditation and biofeedback systems).

INTERVIEWS

- Dr. Andrew Newberg – The value of meditation.

- Dr. Robert Emmons – Enhanced happiness and health by cultivating gratitude.

- Dr. Brett Steenbarger – Achieving peak performance in high-pressure professions.

- Interview with Dr. Andrew Newberg – The value of meditation.

Interview with Dr. Andrew Newberg – The value of meditation.

BACKGROUND:

Dr. Andrew Newberg is an Associate Professor in the Department of Radiology and Psychiatry and Adjunct Assistant Professor in the Department of Religious Studies at the University of Pennsylvania. He has published a variety of neuroimaging studies related to aging and dementia. He has also researched the neurophysiological correlates of meditation, prayer, and how brain function is associated with mystical and religious experiences. In 2009 he published the book *How God Changes the Brain: Breakthrough Findings from a Leading Neuroscientist*, in collaboration with Mark Waldman.

HIGHLIGHTS:

- ⟳ Scientists are researching what elements of meditation may help manage stress and improve memory.

- ⟳ Meditation requires practice and dedication: ongoing research focuses on techniques that would be easier to teach and practice.

MEDITATION MAY HELP MANAGE STRESS AND IMPROVE MEMORY

Dr. Newberg, thank you for being with us today. Can you please explain the source of your interests at the intersection of brain research and spirituality?

Since I was a kid, I had a keen interest in spiritual practice. I always wondered how spirituality and religion affect us, and over time I came to appreciate how science can help us explore and understand the world around us, including why we humans care about spiritual practices. This, of course, led me to be particularly interested in brain research.

During medical school I was particularly attracted by the problem of consciousness. I was fortunate to meet researcher Dr. Eugene D'Aquili in the early 1990s, who had been doing much research on religious practices' effect on the brain since the 1970s. Through him I came to see that brain imaging can provide a fascinating window into the brain.

Can we define religion and spirituality – which sound to me as involving very different brain processes – and why learning about them may be helpful from a purely secular, scientific point of view?

Good point, definitions matter, since different people may be searching for God in different ways. I view being religious as participating in organized rituals and shared beliefs, such as going to church. Being spiritual, on the other hand, is more of an individual practice, whether we call it meditation, or relaxation, or prayer, aimed at expanding the self, developing a sense of oneness with the universe.

What is happening is that specific practices that have traditionally been associated with religious and spiritual contexts may also be very useful from a mainstream, secular, health point of view, beyond those contexts. Scientists are researching, for example, what elements of meditation may help manage stress and improve memory. How breathing and meditation techniques can contribute to health and wellness. For example, my lab is now conducting a study where 15 older adults with memory problems are practicing Kirtan Kriya meditation during 8 weeks, and we have found very promising preliminary outcomes in terms of the impact on brain function. This work is being funded by the Alzheimer's Research and Prevention Foundation, but we have submitted a grant request to the National Institute of Health as well.

Can you give an overview of the benefits of meditation, including Richard Davidson's studies on mindfulness meditation?

There are many types of meditation – and we each are researching different practices – which of course share some common elements, but are different in nature. Dr. Davidson has access to the Dalai Lama and many Buddhist practitioners, so much of his research centers on mindfulness meditation. We have easier access to Franciscan monks and to practitioners of Kirtan Kriya meditation.

At its core, meditation is an active process that requires alertness and attention, which explains why we often find increased brain activity in frontal lobes during practice. Usually you need to focus on something – a mantra, a visual or verbal prompt – while you monitor breathing.

A variety of studies have already shown the stress management benefits of meditation, resulting in what is often called Mindfulness Based Stress Reduction. What we are researching now is what are the cognitive – attention, memory – benefits? It is clear that memory depends on attention and the ability to screen out distractions – so we want to measure the effect of meditation on the brain, both structurally and functionally.

To measure the brain activation patterns we have been using SPECT imaging, which involves injecting small amounts of radioactive tracers in volunteers, and helps us get a better view of what happens during practice (fMRI is much more noisy). To measure functional benefits we use the typical batteries of neuropsychology testing.

MEDITATION IN EVERYDAY LIFE

If there is a growing body of evidence behind the health and cognitive benefits of meditation – what is preventing a more widespread adoption of the practice, perhaps in ways similar to yoga, which is now pretty much a mainstream activity?

Well, the reality is that meditation requires practice and dedication. It is not an easy fix. And some of the best-researched meditation techniques, such as mindfulness meditation, are very intensive. You need a trained facilitator. You need to stick to the practice.

In fact, that's why our ongoing research focused on a much easier to teach and practice technique. We want to see if people can practice on their own, at home, a few minutes a day for a few weeks.

The other problem is that this is not a standardized practice, so there is a lot of confusion: many different meditation techniques, with different sets of priorities and styles.

My advice for interested people would be to look for something simple, easy to try first, ensuring the practice is compatible with one's beliefs and goals. You need to match practice with need: understand the specific goals you have in mind, your schedule and lifestyle, and find something practical. Otherwise, you will not stick to it (similar to people who never show up at the health club despite paying fees).

New York Times columnist David Brooks recently wrote two very thought-provoking articles, one on the Cognitive Age we are living in, another on the Neural Buddhists, where he quotes your work. What is the big picture, the main implications for society from your research?

I believe Philosophy complements Science, and all of us human beings would benefit from spiritual practices to achieve higher state of being, develop compassion, increase awareness, in ways compatible with any religious or secular beliefs. This is the main theme of my book, *How God Changes Brain*: how we develop a shared knowledge of our common biology, and celebrate the differences which are based on our specific contexts. We are spiritual and social beings.

From an education point of view, I believe schools will need to recognize that rote learning is not enough, and add to the mix practices to improve cognition, and manage stress and relationships.

That spiritual angle may prove controversial in a number of scientific quarters. What would you, for example, say to biologist Richard Dawkins (a prominent advocate of atheism and critic of religion)?

I'd tell him that we all view the world through the lens of our brains, reflecting our cultural, social, and personal background. His view is based on his lens. Same as mine. All of us have a belief system. His is not particularly more accurate than everybody else's.

We shouldn't throw out the baby with bathwater. I don't think religion is a black & white matter: yes, fundamentalism is a problem, as is rejecting data and ignoring scientific findings. But there are also good elements: the motivation to care about human beings, to develop compassion, to perfect ourselves and our world.

What is one recent finding or reflection, from your own work or others', that you'd like more people of all ages to know about as they try to maintain/enhance their own brain fitness?

Based on our latest research, we find that one of the most profound ways to improve brain functioning is to change the way we speak and listen to others. Consciousness, the way we become aware of ourselves and reflect on the decisions we make, is shaped in large part by a unique neurological phenomenon known as inner speech. In other words, we have a constant jumble of thoughts flowing into working memory, where we become aware of a very small part of it for a very brief period of time – about 10-20 seconds. Thus, if we want to be able to recall more than a small fraction of what others say, we may want to slow down the overall pace of conversation, and also to do what we can to increase our working memory capacity. And here meditation can be of help — we hypothesize that the combination of concentrated attention combined with music and hand movements while doing the sa-ta-na-ma or Kirtan Kriya meditation that we have studied may contribute to an increase in specific memory functions.

**Interview with Dr. Robert Emmons –
Enhanced happiness and health by cultivating gratitude.**

BACKGROUND:

Prof. Robert Emmons studies gratitude for a living as Professor of Psychology at UC Davis and is Editor-In-Chief of the Journal of Positive Psychology. In 2007, he published "Thanks: How the New Science of Gratitude Can Make You Happier", an interdisciplinary book that provides a research-based synthesis of the topic as well as practical suggestions.

HIGHLIGHTS:

- In the context of positive psychology, taking control of happiness and practicing emotional self-regulation becomes a practical framework to better functioning in life.

- The practice of gratitude can increase happiness levels by around 25%

WHAT IS POSITIVE PSYCHOLOGY?

Prof. Emmons, could you please provide us an overview of the Positive Psychology field so we understand the context for your research?

Sure. Martin Seligman and colleagues launched what was called "positive psychology" in the late 90's as an antidote to the traditional nearly exclusive emphasis of "negative psychology" focused on fixing problems like trauma, addiction, and stress. We want to balance our focus and be able to help everyone, including high-functioning individuals. A number of researchers were investigating the field since the late 80's, but Seligman provided a new umbrella, a new category, with credibility, organized networks and funding opportunities for the whole field.

And where does your own research fit into this overall picture?

I have been researching gratitude for almost 10 years. Gratitude is a positive emotion that has traditionally been the realm of humanists and philosophers, and only recently the subject of a more scientific approach.

We study gratitude not as a merely academic discipline, but as a practical framework to better functioning in life by taking control of happiness levels and practicing the skill of emotional self-regulation.

THE PRACTICE OF GRATITUDE

What are the 3 key messages that you would like readers to take away from your book (see background above)?

First, the practice of gratitude can increase happiness levels by around 25%. Second, this is not hard to achieve – a few hours writing a gratitude journal over 3 weeks can create an effect that lasts 6 months if not more. Third, that cultivating gratitude brings other health effects, such as longer and better quality sleep time.

What are some ways to practice gratitude, and what benefits could we expect? Please refer to your 2003 paper in the Journal of Personality and Social Psychology, where I found fascinating quotes such as that "The ability to notice, appreciate, and savior the elements of one life has been viewed as a crucial element of well-being."

The most common method we use in our research is to ask people to keep a "Gratitude Journal" where you write something you feel grateful for. Doing so 4 times a week, for as little as 3 weeks, is often enough to create a meaningful difference in one level of happiness. Another exercise is to write a "Gratitude Letter" to a person who has exerted a positive influence on one's life but whom we have not properly thanked in the past, and then to meet that person and read the letter to them face to face.

The benefits seem to be very similar using both methods in terms of enhanced happiness, health and wellbeing. Most of the outcomes are self-reported, but there is an increasing emphasis on measuring objective data such as cortisol and stress levels, heart rate variability, and even brain activation patterns. The work of Richard Davidson is exemplary in that respect, showing how mindfulness practice can rewire some activation patterns in the frontal lobes.

Now, let me give an overview of the paper you mention, titled *Counting Blessings versus Burdens: An Experimental Investigation of Gratitude and Subjective Well-Being in Daily Life.* The paper includes 3 separate studies, so I will just be able to provide a quick glimpse. More than a hundred adults were all asked to keep a journal, and were randomly assigned to 3 different groups. Group A had to write about things they felt grateful about. Group B about things they found annoying, irritating. Group C about things that had had a major impact on them. 2 out of the 3 different experiments were relatively intense and short term (keeping a daily journal for 2–3 weeks), while one required a weekly entry during 10 weeks.

Across the 3 different studies we found that people in the gratitude group generally evidenced higher-levels of well-being than those in the comparison conditions, especially when compared to Group B (the one journaling about hassles), but also compared to the "neutral" group.

In the longer study, which ran for 10 weeks, we also saw a positive effect on hours of sleep and on time spent exercising, on more optimistic expectations for the coming week, and fewer reported physical symptoms, such as pain. Additionally, we observed an increase in reported connectedness to other people and in likelihood of helping another person deal with a personal problem.

We could then say that we can train ourselves to develop a more grateful attitude and optimistic outlook in life, resulting in well-being and health improvements, and even in becoming better-not just happier– citizens. And probably one can expect few negative side effects from keeping a gratitude journal. What do you think prevents more people from benefiting from these research findings?

Great question, I reflect often on that. My sense is that some people feel uncomfortable talking about these topics, since they may sound too spiritual, or religious. Others simply don't want to feel obligated to the person who helped them, and never come to realize the boost in energy, enthusiasm, and social benefits that come from a more grateful, connected life.

Judith Beck talked to us recently about her work helping dieters learn important mental skills through cognitive therapy techniques. You talk about gratitude. Other positive psychologists focus on forgiveness. How can we know which of these techniques may be helpful for us?

The key is to reflect on ones goal and current situation. For example, the practice of forgiveness can be most appropriate for people who have high levels of anger and resentment. Cognitive therapy has been shown to be very effective against depression. In a sense both groups are trying to eliminate the negative. Gratitude is different in that it is better suited for highly functioning individuals who simply want to feel better — enhancing the positive.

Interview with Dr. Brett Steenbarger – Achieving peak performance in high-pressure professions.

BACKGROUND:

The applications of cognitive neuroscience to trading and finance are central to Dr. Brett Steenbarger's research. Dr. Steenbarter wears many hats, including Associate Professor of Psychiatry and Behavioral Sciences at SUNY Upstate Medical University, active trader of over 30 years, former Director of Trader Development for Kingstree Trading, LLC, and author of *The Psychology of Trading: Tools and Techniques for Minding the Markets* and the recent *Enhancing Trader Performance: Proven Strategies From the Cutting Edge of Trading Psychology*. He writes feature columns for the Trading Markets website and several trading publications, including Stocks Futures and Options.

HIGHLIGHTS:

- Traders would benefit from following the example of elite performers and have many tools at their disposal – including books, simulation programs, biofeedback programs for emotional management, and coaches.

- Many people who do not end up performing at a high level are not motivated to follow the same level of intensive and systematic training as elite performers.

WHAT TRADERS AND OTHER PROFESSIONALS CAN LEARN FROM ELITE PERFORMERS

Give us some context on your interest in trading performance and how it led you to your new book.

My main interest is how to enhance cognitive and emotional development among traders to help them become more successful. My first book, *The Psychology of Trading*, focused on emotional and stress management, and tried to help traders – both professionals and amateurs – overcome the emotional disruptions of trading. My new book, Enhancing Trader Performance, helps traders develop their own training programs or, we may even call them, "brain gyms," to build their skills, strengthen their mental capacities, and improve their performance.

What is the premise of your new book, Enhancing Trader Performance?

The premise is that elite performers in highly competitive fields share common traits. This includes people in such fields as athletics, performing arts, chess, the military, and medicine. I review the research regarding what makes people successful in those fields, find the common factors behind their success, and then apply the findings to traders.

What are those common factors for top performers? And what differentiates elite performers from the rest?

The elite performers are most distinguished by the structure of their learning process. From a relatively early age, they are engaged in an intensive learning process that builds upon their natural talents. They find a niche – a field that makes use of their talents – and become absorbed by a deliberative and systematic learning process that provides them with continuous feedback about their performance.

The recipe for success seems to be talent, skill, hard work, and opportunity. In contrast, many people who do not end up performing at a high level are driven mostly by practical reasons to enter a given field and are not motivated to follow the same level of intensive and systematic training as the elite performers.

What type of training and practice will help traders function at peak performance levels?

Traders typically devote little time to practice and a structured learning process. I want to encourage them to see that "learning on the job" is not a substitute for breaking down skills into components, drilling these, receiving feedback about performance, and making continuous modifications and improvements.

In every field, elite performers devote more time to practice than to the actual performance. To perform at the highest level, you need to protect and optimize practice and learning time. The average trader does not do that, and the result is that many traders lose their trading capital within seven months of trading. To develop themselves, I suggest traders structure their learning processes.

There are several elements to this development:

○ Simulation and Biofeedback Tools: There are very good simulations out there that can help traders become more sensitive to patterns in the market and internalize these. The ability to play and replay market days provides traders with enhanced screen time to accelerate and deepen learning. Another set of tools includes biofeedback programs that help traders manage their emotions. Biofeedback is especially helpful in reducing emotional arousal that can disrupt executive functions such as judgment, planning, analyzing, and reasoning.

○ Reflection and Regular Feedback: Traders who utilize programs to provide them with metrics on their trading performance – analyses of their winning and losing trades – have considerable data at their disposal. The patterns revealed by these metrics help traders figure out both strengths and weaknesses. Many times, building on successes is more important than trying to change weaknesses. Constant feedback on trading results shows traders what they do best – and help them do more of it.

○ Role of Mentors and Coaches: In many performance fields, such as music and tennis, coaches help students break down their performance into component skills and then systematically work on these individually and in combination. The mentor is someone who can structure the learning process for the developing performer and help them move along the path from being a novice to being competent to being expert. Both are useful for traders.

Interesting analogy. Who would be a good "trader coach" and where does one find one?

Ideally, you need an experienced and successful trader who is familiar with the kind of trading that you will be doing. The book contains an appendix with different resources that can help traders find educational and mentoring resources. For emotional development, traders can also coach themselves with practical cognitive and behavioral techniques and build new, positive ways of thinking and behaving. The last two chapters of the book provide readers with self-help manuals for utilizing these techniques.

What are the key components of top performance in trading, and what skills traders can develop?

First, we must differentiate between short-term and long-term traders. For short-term traders, the priority is the ability to process large amounts of information and to quickly see patterns that will lead to effective decision making. They need speed, and good working memory. For long-term traders, analytical skills are paramount.

For both, I would add, knowing how to deal with "the emotional factor" is very important. Many traders get very frustrated when their bets do not go the way they expected, and become paralyzed or make nonlogical decisions. Others may lose concentration and focus when they get fatigued, and make impulsive decisions. But I would stress that there is more to trading success than controlling emotions. It takes talent, skill, and a constant learning process.

I would also emphasize that, yes, we can train and get better at many things, but it is equally important to ensure an optimal fit between our trading talents and interests: the markets we trade and the ways we trade them. There has to be a fit between what we're good at and the opportunities afforded by a particular market and trading style.

How applicable are these findings to professionals in other fields?

People who aspire to be top performers in any field must build on what comes naturally to them, in order to be truly motivated and absorb constant learning. They will need to structure programs to develop their skills and work these programs diligently. Because elite performers do what comes naturally, they become absorbed in the development of their skills. If you have to motivate yourself to work at something, it is probably not your calling.

BRAIN TRAINING PROGRAMS:
NOW AND IN THE FUTURE

What training programs are available today and which ones do you foresee will be available in the future?

First, I find that Dr. Elkhonon Goldberg's metaphor of a gymnasium for the brain is very appealing. We will be seeing more and more tools for cognitive and brain fitness. Dr. Goldberg cites considerable research that indicates we can improve the functioning of our frontal cortex – home of our executive functions such as reasoning, planning, judgment, analysis, and problem-solving – through structured exercises, much as we can build muscles in the gym.

Today, traders have very realistic simulation programs that can help them identify market patterns and improve decision making. True, as Professor Gopher said in your interview with him, what matters is the cognitive fidelity of those simulations, and how they will help traders see new, non-historical, patterns. But, at the very least, existing simulation packages help traders learn very quickly how to identify a wealth of recurring patterns in markets.

Finally, I work with many traders on their emotional reactions – especially new traders. Behavioral techniques can be very helpful to develop calmer, open minds and good attitudes. In a blog post, I stress the need to keep an open mind and avoid missing unexpected "gorillas" in the market. We need to be aware of and manage the narrowing of our attention that usually follows hyper-focus. For the many people out there who become angry and frustrated after trading losses, I recommend exercises such as deep breathing and visual imagery, which, after a period of practice, can be applied very quickly to our work when we need it. These techniques can be reinforced by the use of biofeedback programs that provide real-time visual feedback on a trader's "internal performance." The biofeedback programs reveal whether traders are in the zone of optimal learning and performance or are becoming too stressed, anxious, and impulsive.

It is important to understand the role of emotions: they are not "bad". They are very useful signals. It is, however, important to become aware of them to avoid being engulfed by them, and to learn how to manage them.

What is one recent finding or reflection, from your own work or others', that you'd like more people of all ages to know about as they try to maintain/enhance their own brain fitness?

My primary work is with investors and traders in the financial markets. They deal with stress, risk, and uncertainty on a daily basis and yet need to stay calm and focused in order to make the best decisions possible. A recent book by John Coates, *The Hour Between Dog and Wolf*, nicely summarizes the evidence that the inner workings of our brains and bodies affect how we think, feel, and behave. The challenge for maintaining and extending brain fitness is, in part, the challenge of overcoming our biological heritage: it is not always prudent to attack or flee when our bodies are in fight or flight mode. By placing ourselves in simulated emergency scenarios (through visualization and guided imagery, through hypnosis, through actual constructed simulations) and rehearsing optimal modes of responding, we can cultivate resilience during the most challenging of situations. While this is of clear relevance to people in such professions as investment management, firefighting, the military, police work, and athletics, such training can also help us deal better with life's daily challenges, from parenting to handling work conflicts. Bottom line: think of life as a gymnasium and the obstacles we encounter as the weights we must lift to get stronger. When you can view challenges as resources toward development and not as unfortunate obstacles to be avoided, you'll be well along the path toward brain fitness.

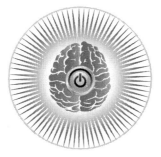

CHAPTER 8

CROSS-TRAIN YOUR BRAIN

In a modern society we are confronted too with a wide range of increasingly abstract and interconnected problems. Successfully dealing with such an environment requires a highly fit brain, capable of adapting to new situations and challenges throughout life. Consequently, we expect cross-training the brain to soon become as mainstream as cross-training the body is today, going beyond unstructured mental activity in order to maximize specific brain functions. The goal of this chapter is to help you navigate the growing field of brain training techniques and tools.

WHAT IS BRAIN TRAINING?

We can define brain training as the structured and efficient use of mental exercises designed to build targeted brain-based networks and capacities. Its aim is to improve specific brain functions, similar to physical conditioning training. Since "neurons that fire together wire together" (see Chapter 1), repeatedly stimulating (i.e. training) a specific network of neurons results in new and strengthened connections in this network. This in turn translates into improved neuronal efficiency that can result in better and more sustained performance.

How is brain training different from mental stimulation?

As discussed before, anything we do involving novelty, variety, and challenge stimulates the brain and can contribute to building capacity and brain reserve. For instance, learning how to play the piano activates a number of brain functions (attention, memory, motor skills, etc.), which triggers changes in the underlying neuronal networks. Indeed, musicians have larger brain volume in areas that are important for playing an instrument: motor, auditory and visuospatial regions. However, we need to recognize that such an activity may take thousands of hours before paying off in terms of brain fitness. It constitutes a great and pleasurable mental effort, and helps build cognitive reserve, but it is different by nature from more targeted and efficient brain training interventions. To take an analogy from the world of physical fitness, you can try to stay fit by playing pickup soccer games (an active leisure activity, certainly better than watching a documentary about soccer) AND by putting effort towards training specific muscle groups and capacities such as cardio endurance, abdominal muscles, and thigh muscle.

Under what conditions can brain training work?

This is the million dollar question. Evidence is growing that brain training can work. The question remains, however, of how to maximize one's chances of success and maximize the likelihood of transfer from training to daily life.

As mentioned earlier, the best reference to date to compare the value of brain training vs. dozens of other alternatives is the extensive NIH meta-analysis released in 2010. Its conclusion was that cognitive training showed a small protective effect, just as physical activity did. Importantly, the level of evidence for this result was rated as high, meaning that a clear effect was present.

Why do we still often hear that brain training does not work? Because of the different understandings of what "brain training" and "work" mean. A machine to train abdominal muscles probably won't "work" if what we measure is blood pressure. A "plane" won't fly if it wasn't a "plane" to start with, but a donkey.

An important aspect to look at when evaluating whether a brain training method or program works is the extent to which the training effects "transfer" to untrained tasks and to benefits in daily life. We know from common experience that practice usually triggers improvement in the practiced task. For instance, by practicing meditation one can be expected to get better at meditating. The more important requirement is to show that this improvement transfers to other, untrained, tasks, ideally activities performed in everyday life. This would show that the overall cognitive abilities targeted by the technique were indeed trained.

Building on an analysis of documented examples of brain training techniques that "work" or "transfer," as well as extensive discussions held at the 2011 and 2012 SharpBrains Virtual Summits, we suggest the following five conditions need to be met for brain training to be likely to translate into meaningful real world improvements:

1. Training must engage and exercise a core brain-based capacity or neural circuit identified to be relevant to real-life outcomes. Noteworthy examples include executive attention, working memory, speed of processing and emotional regulation, as well as others discussed throughout the interviews with scientists in this book. Many supposed "brain training" games fail to provide any actual "brain training" because they were never properly designed to target specific and relevant brain functions.

2. The training must target a performance bottleneck – otherwise it is an exercise in vanity similar to building the largest biceps in town while neglecting the rest of the body. A critical question to ask is: Which brain function do I need to optimize? With physical fitness, effective training begins with a target in mind: Is the goal to train abdominal muscles? Biceps? Cardio capacity? So it goes for brain fitness, where the question becomes: Is the goal to optimize driving-related cognitive skills? Concentration? Memory? Regulating stress and emotions? The choice of a technique or technology should be driven

by your goal. For instance, if you need to train your executive functions but use a program designed to enhance speed of processing, you may well conclude that this program does not "work." But this program may work for somebody whose bottleneck is speed of processing (as often happens in older adults).

3. A minimum "dose" of 15 hours total per targeted brain function, performed over 8 weeks or less, is necessary for real improvement. Training only a few hours across a wide variety of brain functions, such as in the "BBC brain training" experiment, should not be expected to trigger real-world benefits, in the same way that going to the gym a couple times per month and doing an assortment of undirected exercises cannot be expected to result in increased muscle strength and physical fitness.

4. Training must be adaptive to performance, require effortful attention, and increase in difficulty. This is a key advantage of software-based "brain training" over pen-and-paper-based activities. Think about the number of hours you have spent doing crossword or Sudoku puzzles, or mastering any new subject for that matter, in a way that was either too easy for you and became boring or way too difficult and became frustrating. Interactive, automated training has the capacity to constantly monitor your level of performance and adapt accordingly.

5. Over the long-term, the key is continued practice for continued benefits. Just as you wouldn't expect to derive lifelong benefits from running a few hours this month, and then not exercising ever again, you shouldn't expect lifelong benefits from a one-time brain training activity. Remember that "cells that fire together wire together" – while the minimum dose described above may act as a threshold to start seeing some benefits, continued practice, either at a reduced number of hours or as a periodic "booster," is a final condition for transfer to real-world benefits over time.

THE CASE FOR CROSS-TRAINING

The circumstances and goals of each person influences what brain functions to train. For instance, if the intended user is a busy and often stressed-out executive, he or she may want to focus on managing stress and building emotional resilience. If the user is a driver in his or her 60's, improving speed-of-processing and so-called Useful Field of View (a predictor of driving safety) may be a better start.

Age must also enter into the equation when assessing what skills need to be trained. As discussed in Chapter 1, the brain changes as we age: some functions tend to improve, some decline. The frontal lobes support what scientists call executive functions, which include abilities such as adapting to new situations and planning and, as we age, the frontal lobes may need extra work to increase neuroprotection.

In the absence of widely available and reliable assessments to pinpoint your bottlenecks, and in the absence of standardized and well-validated brain training approaches, we believe the most reasonable approach is to start by cross-training using research-based and time-efficient methodologies.

Let's now review the four core research-based brain training methodologies.

MEDITATION TO TRAIN EMOTIONAL RESPONSES AND ATTENTIONAL FOCUS

You may be wondering what meditation has to do with brain training. In fact, as described in Chapter 7 and below, meditation has been shown to improve specific cognitive functions such as emotional regulation and attention. As such it can be considered a brain training technique – perhaps even the original one.

Styles of meditation differ. As discussed in the previous chapter, some techniques use concentration and mantras, while others rely on body relaxation, breathing practice, and mental imagery. Since mindfulness meditation is among the most used and studied type of meditation, we will mostly focus on it. Mindfulness refers to a process that leads to a mental state characterized by a non-judgmental awareness of the present experience (one's thoughts and sensations as well as the environment).

There are two major brain functions that can be enhanced via mindfulness meditation, one having to do with emotion and the other with attention. Practicing mindfulness meditation can indeed help train us to better control our emotions, and stress in particular. For instance, a recent meta-analysis of 39 studies looking at over 1,000 participants who received mindfulness-based therapy for a range of conditions (from cancer to depression) showed that mindfulness meditation was effective for improving anxiety and mood symptoms. (For a more comprehensive review of meditation as a brain training technique to manage stress and build resilience, please see Chapter 7.)

Practicing mindfulness meditation can also help train the ability to control your focus of attention, to keep it on the task at hand while ignoring distractions. Indeed, numerous studies compared people who practice meditation to people who do not, and found that the first group showed enhanced attentional processes. The problem with many of these studies is that subjects in the two groups may differ along numerous dimensions to start with. The benefits observed in the group practicing meditation could be due to other things.

Better controlled studies, in which a group of non-meditators is trained to meditate and compared to an untrained naïve group, support the beneficial effects of meditation on attentional control. For instance, Michael Posner and his colleagues randomly assigned participants to either Integrative Body-Mind Training (IBMT) or to relaxation training for a 2007 study. Both programs lasted 5 days, with 20 minutes of training per day. IBMT is a meditation technique developed in China in the 1990's. It stresses a balanced state of relaxation while focusing attention. Thought control is achieved with the help of a coach through posture, relaxation, body-mind harmony, and balance. The results of this study showed that after training, participants in the IBMT training group showed more improvement in a task measuring executive attention than the control group. The IBMT training also helped reduce cortisol levels caused by mental stress. In 2010, the same team of researchers replicated this study while also scanning the 45 participants' brains. IBMT training resulted in changes in the neuronal connections involving the anterior cingulate, a brain area related to the ability to regulate emotions and behavior. Eleven hours of meditation training was sufficient to trigger changes in a brain area related to self-regulation – and this "dose" is consistent with the minimum 10-15 hours per targeted brain function suggested above for successful training.

Recently, a study showed that a Mindfulness Based Stress Reduction (MBSR) program could also change the structure of the brain. Participants in the program meditated for 30 minutes per day for 8 weeks. At the end of the training, the brains of trained participants showed changes that were not present in the non-trained participants' brains. Gray matter was thicker in several parts of the brain involved in learning, memory, empathy and emotional regulation, suggesting that meditation may change the efficiency of these brain functions.

IBMT and MBSR do seem to improve attentional focus. Is this true of all types of meditation? Not all have been tested but it is likely: the key seems to be to focus on a specific stimulus while meditating and being able to control this focus. For example, you can read Dr. Newberg's interview in the prior chapter on the benefits of Kirtan Kriya meditation, which is particularly intriguing given its light protocol of only 12-minutes per day.

In sum, there is evidence that meditating can increase our attentional control, and this is a critical factor in optimizing brain health and performance. As Andrew Newberg (whose interview you can find at the end of the previous chapter) highlights: "It is clear that memory depends on attention and the ability to screen out distractions."

Here is Dr. Newberg's advice if you are ready to give meditation a try: "There is a lot of confusion: many different meditation techniques, with different sets of priorities and styles. My advice for interested people would be look for something simple, easy to try first, ensuring the practice is compatible with one's beliefs and goals. You need to match practice with need: understand the specific goals you have in mind, your schedule and lifestyle, and find something practical. Otherwise, you will not stick to it (similar to people who never show up at the health club despite paying fees)."

REFRAMING THOUGHT PROCESSES
VIA COGNITIVE BEHAVIORAL THERAPY

Cognitive therapy (CT) is a type of Cognitive Behavioral Therapy (CBT) founded by Dr. Aaron Beck. It is based on the idea that the way people perceive their experience influences their behaviors and emotions. The therapist teaches the patient cognitive and behavioral skills to modify his or her dysfunctional thinking and actions. CT aims at improving specific traits, behaviors, or cognitive skills, such as planning and flexibility, which are executive functions. As such it can be considered a brain training methodology. CT has been shown to be effective in many contexts, such as depression, high levels of anxiety, insomnia, obsessive-compulsive disorder, and phobias.

Neuroimaging has been used to demonstrate the effects of CT on the brain. Let's take the example of spider phobia. In 2003, Vincent Paquette and his colleagues showed that before the cognitive therapy, the fear induced by viewing film clips depicting spiders was correlated with significant activation of specific brain areas, such as the amygdala. After the intervention was completed (one three-hour group session per week, for four weeks), viewing the same spider films did not provoke activation of those areas. Dr. Judith Beck, Dr. Aaron Beck's daughter, explains that the adults in this study were able to "train their brains" which resulted in reducing the stress response triggered by spiders.

So CT seems effective in dealing with several clinical issues. What about the use of CT to help healthy individual change unwanted though processes? Recently, Dr. Judith Beck has successfully used CT to help dieters acquire new skills in order to achieve their goals (see Dr. Beck's interview at the end of this Chapter). According to Dr. Beck the main message of CT and its application in the diet world is that problems losing weight are not the dieter's fault. These problems reflect a lack of skills, which can be acquired through training. What skills is Dr. Beck talking about? Mostly executive functions: the skills to plan in advance, to motivate oneself, to monitor one's behavior, etc.

In 2005, researchers conducted a randomized controlled study confirming the effect of CT on weight loss. Nearly all 65 participants completed the program, and the short-term intervention (10-week, 30-hours) showed a significant long-term weight reduction, even larger (when compared to the 40 individuals in the control group) after 18 months than right after the 10-week program.

COGNITIVE TRAINING TO OPTIMIZE TARGETED BRAIN FUNCTIONS

For many years, neuropsychologists have helped individuals suffering from a variety of brain injuries relearn how to talk, walk or make decisions. Among other tools, cognitive exercises (including computer-assisted strategies) have been used to retrain the compromised abilities. A variety of commercial programs are now making cognitive training available to the general public via online and/or mobile applications, presenting major opportunities—and challenges.

We define "cognitive training" as fully-automated applications designed to assess and enhance targeted cognitive functions. Adaptive, technology-based programs offer the user various tools to exercise different brain structures and cognitive skills by continually responding to performance and increasing the difficulty level incrementally. These programs can be delivered either online or via smart phone and tablets, and sometimes required specific hardware elements. They can be either sold directly to consumers or offered only under clinical supervision.

Are they effective?

Let's first dissect why the systematic 2010 NIH meta-analysis found cognitive training to be a protective factor against cognitive decline. When evaluating the role of cognitive training, one of the major studies reviewed was the five years ACTIVE study conducted by Willis and her colleagues. This study was one of the first large randomized controlled trials ever published in the area of cognitive training. The several thousand participants in this groundbreaking study were 73.6 years old on average. They were exposed to various forms of mental training: reasoning, memory and speed training. The training of processing speed was computer-based. Participants showed an improvement in the skills trained and a narrow transfer to non-trained tasks, and retained a significant percentage of this improvement when tested five years later. The group who received the training in processing speed showed the most pronounced short-term and long-term improvements. Based on a review of the numerous publications that came out of this study, the 2010 NIH analysis concluded that cognitive training confers a modest but consistent benefit on cognitive functions and can be considered protective against cognitive decline. While far from a panacea, it is noteworthy that an intervention which only took 10 hours in Year 1 still resulted in measurable benefits 5 years later.

Since the publication of the ACTIVE study, a growing number of randomized controlled studies have shown how well-directed cognitive training programs can produce cognitive and other improvements to daily life. At the same time, other studies have found no such benefits, and much controversy has surrounded the specific marketing claims made by a number of companies in the field. Here we are reminded of Aristotle's saying, "Virtue is the mean between two vices." It is important neither to fall for misleading and exaggerated marketing claims, nor to throw the baby out with the bathwater and miss out on opportunities available today.

One computerized program, Brain Fitness Classic by Posit Science (a precursor to brainHQ, discussed later in this chapter), underwent testing in the IMPACT (Improvement in Memory with Plasticity-based Adaptive Cognitive Training) study conducted by Dr. Elizabeth Zelinski (see her interview at the end of Chapter 4). Participants were 487 dementia-free individuals, 65 years old and over. Half of the participants used the 6 brain exercises included in the computerized program one hour per day, five days per week, for eight weeks (40 hours total). The other half spent the same amount of time using computers to view educational programs on history, art, and literature, and received quizzes after each session. Participants in the training group improved at the trained tasks. Interestingly, their performance on standardized measures of memory and attention also improved, suggesting some level of transfer of benefits. A 2011 study reported the 3-month follow-up results of this intervention, showing that, 3 months after the initial training, most of the improvement observed in the training group was still present, although not as strongly. In other words, without reinforcement, the cognitive training effect was maintained but waned over time. This suggests that regular training is needed for longer lasting benefits.

There are a variety of programs, some commercially-available some not, aimed at improving working memory (WM). Working memory is the memory system that allows you to hold information briefly in mind for the purpose of the task at hand. In 2005, Torkel Klingberg and his colleagues conducted a randomized controlled study to test whether the use of Cogmed working memory training could help improve WM performance in children with attention-deficit/hyperactivity disorder (ADHD). The training period was at least 20 days. Results showed that training WM using Cogmed increased the performance of the children in untrained tasks measuring WM as well as in tasks measuring response inhibition and complex reasoning. The benefits were still present when the children were tested again 3 month after the training. Since 2005, multiple other studies conducted by independent scientists have shown a variety of benefits from using Cogmed with children and teenagers with ADHD and with patients with brain injury, and possibly with older adults. Another protocol to enhance working memory involves the so-called n-dual task, and you can read the interview with Dr. Martin Buschkuehl at the end of this chapter to learn more about this intervention.

Two recent studies show that the benefits of cognitive training can sometimes transfer to unexpected aspects of behavior. For instance, a 2010 study took the ACTIVE data and looked at the effect of the training on the participants' personal control or sense of control. It was found that the reasoning and speed of processing training resulted in an improvement in the sense of control. Why might this be? The authors reasoned that this was because the training focused on maintaining or improving older adults' cognitive abilities, which preserved their independence during a period of their lives when cognitive abilities and performance are usually declining. Another recent study showed that training inductive reasoning skills for 16 weeks enhanced openness to new experiences in older adults, a personality trait that was thought to be relatively fixed.

Much research is underway to better understand the cognitive training conditions and factors that may result in measurable long-term health benefits, and to distinguish between substantive and baseless claims. As Dr. Jerry Edwards (whose interview can be found at the end of this chapter) points out: "It is too early to say whether we can really reverse decline in a permanent way. There are many skills involved and the studies are not long enough to really compare different trajectories."

In sum, a growing body of evidence suggests that many brain functions which were thought to be fixed, such as working memory, are actually trainable; that "old dogs can learn new tricks" and still work on improving cognition in their 60's, 70's, and beyond; and that transfer of benefits to untrained tasks, while not easy, is possible. This may not sound like much, but it represents a significant leap from only 20 years ago, when most scientists would have probably said that the adult brain has no capacity for plasticity and that brain functions are therefore un-trainable, so what is the point of even trying.

BIOFEEDBACK TO MONITOR AND ENHANCE PHYSIOLOGICAL RESPONSES

In the previous chapter we discussed several lifestyle-based options to regulate stress and develop emotional resilience. Another option, which can properly be considered to be brain training given its structure and efficiency, is by using biofeedback products. Biofeedback hardware devices can measure and display various physiological variables such as skin conductivity and heart rate variability, helping users learn to be self-aware and to self-adjust. The basic technology has been used for decades in medicine and has only recently emerged as reasonably-priced applications for consumers. It can provide a great complement to meditation since it adds a feedback loop to better self-monitor and refine the impact of the practice.

Neurofeedback is a type of biofeedback relying specifically on electrophysiological measures of brain activity. Using electroencephalography (EEG) biofeedback to measure brain waves gives the user feedback on different "mental states," like alertness or relaxation. Despite the growing availability of relatively inexpensive, consumer-directed EEG-devices, we believe that neurofeedback is still a brain training tool mostly useful in research and clinical contexts. We expect that to change soon, once there is more solid data on what specific and standardized protocols benefit mainstream, healthy users.

In contrast, and for the time being, biofeedback based on heart rate variability (HRV) has the support of a more developed evidence base, and devices are becoming quite inexpensive, making them a more obvious starting point.

As described in the previous chapter, heart rate variability (HRV) provides information regarding both PNS and SNS activity. These two systems antagonistically influence the lengths of time between consecutive heartbeats. Faster heart rates, which can be due to increased SNS activity, correspond to a shorter interbeat interval, while slower heart rates have a longer interbeat interval, which can be attributed to increased PNS activity. As such HRV can be viewed as a non-invasive measurement of emotion regulation.

HRV biofeedback products can help users influence their HRV by self-monitoring and self-regulating their breathing, and often come with game-like exercises to help master the core techniques to do so. Knowing how to regulate one's breathing can then become a learned skill, and can in turn help in optimizing brain functions. As an example, Dr. Steenbarger, whose interview can be found at the end of this chapter, recommends the use of relaxation coupled with biofeedback programs to improve a trader's performance. These programs provide real-time visual feedback on a "trader's internal performance." You may be wondering how this may help a trader. It is because of the close relationship between emotion and cognition: emotion strongly affects cognition. Stress, as we mentioned earlier, can be very detrimental to performance. Thus, in jobs where stress can run high it is very important to learn how to self-regulate emotionally in order to improve cognitive and job performance.

TOP BRAIN TRAINING PROGRAMS, BASED ON SHARPBRAINS' ANALYSIS AND SURVEY

When it comes to brain training, there is tremendous variation in what the interventions are designed to do, how much evidence there is to back them up, and how beneficial they seem to be when used outside laboratory environments. This wide variation is often confusing for potential users and even for experts. In the first edition of this book, published in 2009, we tried to offer a snapshot of the wide array of available options, and discussed 21 different products. For this second edition, based on feedback from many readers, we have geared our approach away from an a theoretical discussion of the science behind each and every product and instead towards clear and simple guidance about some "reasonable starting points." Our intention is to provide practical information for those interested in complementing other lifestyle options with a self-directed, technology-based program, not to provide a detailed, comprehensive overview of the entire marketplace (for those interested, SharpBrains released in January 2013 a comprehensive market report titled *"The Digital Brain Health Market 2012–2020: Web-based, mobile and biometrics-based technology to assess, monitor and enhance cognition and brain functioning"*).

Out of the hundreds of products making brain training claims, we are going to highlight only a few that meet strict criteria indicative of high-quality and value to the user. We believe "reasonable starting points" must meet 3 criteria:

1. a well-articulated scientific rationale, and at least a basic and growing level of scientific testing (Research Momentum);

2. sustained growth among a wide variety of users (Market Momentum); and

3. higher-than-average levels of satisfaction among users with the results they have seen (Results Seen).

Assessments of for the first two criteria emerged from the market research analysis performed for SharpBrains' 2013 report *The Digital Health Market 2012-2020,* mentioned above, for which we identified 5 Market Leaders and 10 Companies to Watch, based on their Research and Market Momentum. 185 companies were assessed against eight sub-criteria, as follows:

1. Research Momentum
   - Composition of Scientific Advisory Board
   - Quality of research methodology and framework
   - Publication of direct clinical evidence in peer-reviewed journals
   - Pipeline of clinical trials which involve the companies' products

2. Market Momentum
   - Company revenue, including both absolute numbers and annual growth
   - Amount and type of corporate funding
   - Type and depth of distribution partnerships
   - Level and quality of public support from customers

Next we compiled and analyzed the results from an extensive survey conducted in March/April of 2012 among subscribers of SharpBrains' monthly eNewsletter, designed to elicit feedback from early-adopters and professionals in the field. Among the over 3,000 respondents, more than 1,000 identified at least one brain training product they had used (for themselves or for someone else) and answered several questions on a 5-point scale (from "strongly disagree" to "strongly agree"). A key question was whether people agreed or disagreed with the statement "I have seen the results I wanted," and we identified the 10 companies whose products ranked highest in that question. These responses were the source for our evaluation of the third criterion, Results Seen.

What did we find as a result of this analysis? Only four companies met all three criteria: Research Momentum, Market Momentum, and Results Seen. They are (in alphabetical order):

- Cogmed
- HeartMath

- Lumos Labs
- Posit Science

Before we go ahead and discuss these companies' brain training offerings, though, let's take a moment to dissect some fascinating results from the 2012 SharpBrains Market Survey (analyzed with more granularity in the market report mentioned above).

Results from the 2012 SharpBrains Market Survey

First, these were the most popular brain training programs identified by respondents in our survey:

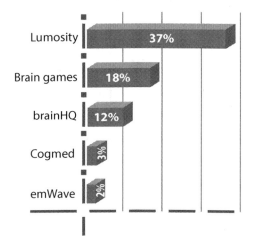

TABLE 3. Most popular brain training products (SharpBrains survey)

As you can see, Lumos Labs' online offering (lumosity.com) seems to have gained significant growth. Posit Science's programs (grouped under new name brainHQ in the charts), no longer aided by PBS-related programming and advertising, maintain a solid user base, and Cogmed and emWave by Heartmath appear to rely on smaller user bases. Again, we would like to emphasize that these numbers represent usage among the early-adopters and professionals that account for the majority of the 45,000+ subscribers to SharpBrains' monthly eNewsletter, rather than the general population at large.

Then we asked survey respondents to answer five questions on a 5-point scale (from "Strongly Disagree" to "Strongly Agree," including a "Neutral" for people who neither agreed nor disagreed) regarding the specific product they had used. For clarity we show the combined "Agree" and "Strongly Agree" results.

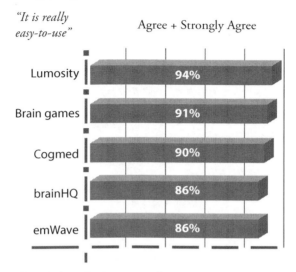

TABLE 4a. Ease of use (SharpBrains survey)

Most products seem easy to use, with Lumosity taking the lead.

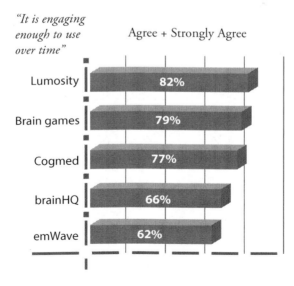

TABLE 4b. Engaging over time (SharpBrains survey)

Here too Lumosity takes a (more narrow) lead. Two of the more targeted products (Posit Science and HeartMath's) don't seem as engaging to use over time.

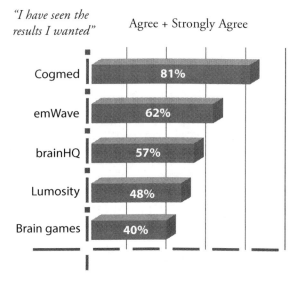

"I have seen the results I wanted" — Agree + Strongly Agree

- Cogmed: 81%
- emWave: 62%
- brainHQ: 57%
- Lumosity: 48%
- Brain games: 40%

TABLE 4c. Desired results seen

Of course, the whole purpose of brain training is to actually see the results you wanted to see when purchasing the product. We worded the question in that way to better enable us to compare diverse expectations and beliefs. Cogmed's working memory training program ranks highest here, followed by HeartMath's and Posit Science's, while "brain games" in general lag behind. It is important to note that these results are better overall than they may seem, since the most common alternative to Strongly Agree or Agree was neither Strongly Disagree nor Disagree, but people who chose to stay Neutral.

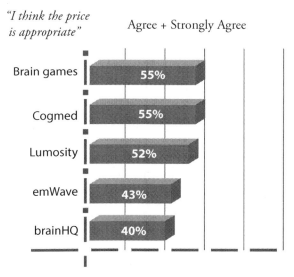

"*I think the price is appropriate*" Agree + Strongly Agree

Brain games	55%
Cogmed	55%
Lumosity	52%
emWave	43%
brainHQ	40%

TABLE 4d. Appropriateness of price

What surprised us the most here is that level of agreement is not perfectly correlated with price itself, but with perception of value and with other alternatives the user may have in mind: Cogmed ranks ahead, with 55% users agreeing with "price is appropriate," while being offered as a service with a cost of over $1,500 by a network of certified providers. Posit Science's low scores may be better now, as the company recently stopped selling its up-to-$400 software products and instead offers a $14/month online subscription.

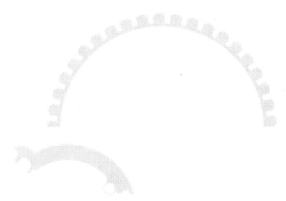

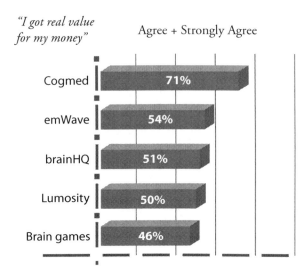

"I got real value for my money"   Agree + Strongly Agree

Cogmed	71%
emWave	54%
brainHQ	51%
Lumosity	50%
Brain games	46%

TABLE 4e. Value for money

Finally, we asked whether respondents thought that they had got real value for their money. All four identified products rated better than general "brain games."

In summary, there is not one single obvious way to answer the question "which is the best brain training product." The answer depends on what you are looking for, your priorities, and your budget. While we do not endorse any product, we feel confident in suggesting that any of these options may make sense as "reasonable starting point."

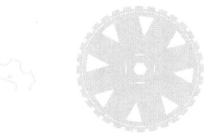

Product Overviews

Let's now take a brief look at each of these offerings.

Product	Target Users	Primary Brain Function/s Targeted	Brief Description	Price
Lumosity, from Lumos Labs www.lumosity.com	All ages	Wide range of cognitive functions	Online cognitive training platform with 30+ exercises. User can personalize training, access quick assessments, and compare performance to other users of the same age to identify strengths and weaknesses.	$9.95/month or $79.95/year
emWave Desktop, from HeartMath www.heartmathstore.com	All ages	Emotional regulation	Combines a software program, biofeedback sensors that measure heart rate variability (HRV), and game-like exercises, to help the user learn how to adjust breathing patterns to regulate stress and emotional coherence.	$249
Cogmed Working Memory Training, from Cogmed www.cogmed.com	Children and adults with a working memory bottleneck	Working memory	Software-based service typically used in educational or clinical settings to help address working memory deficits, often associated with attention deficits, brain injury or normal aging. The program trains working memory, the ability to hold information in mind for a short period of time.	Around $1,500, which includes 5-week training supervised by a certified clinician
brainHQ, from Posit Science www.brainhq.com www.positscience.com	50+ adults	Visual and auditory information processing	Online cognitive training platform with 15+ exercises that integrate the three CD-ROM products previously offered by Posit Science. Primarily aimed at adults who feel it difficult to follow conversations in noisy environments, notice a loss of concentration, or want to maintain safe driving.	$14/month or $96/year

TABLE 5. Top Brain Training Products.

SHARPBRAINS' CHECKLIST FOR EVALUATING BRAIN FITNESS CLAIMS

As mentioned, the programs discussed above are but "reasonable starting points." We are sure many readers are currently considering other options, or may do so in the future. Evaluating the brain fitness claims for a company's products depends on many variable factors, such as the goals, priorities, starting point, and budget of the intended user, which is why there is no general ranking of products that would satisfy everybody. Instead, we have developed a Brain Fitness Evaluation Checklist. When evaluating any product making brain fitness claims we recommend asking the following 10 questions:

1. **Are there credible, university-based scientists (ideally neuropsychologists or cognitive neuroscientists) in the company's scientific advisory board?** Neuropsychologists and cognitive neuroscientists specialize in measuring and understanding human cognition and brain structure and function.

2. **Are there peer-reviewed, scientific papers that have been published in mainstream scientific and professional journals that analyze the effects of the specific product? How many? With what population of users?** This is important to validate the effectiveness and relevance of a particular program.

3. **Does the program tell me which specific brain function(s) I am exercising? What are the specific benefits claimed for using this program?** Some programs present the benefits in such an imprecise way that it is impossible to tell if they will have any results or not. "Exercise your brain" itself is a very vague claim, because activities like gardening or learning a new language provide brain exercise too. You need to see something more specific, like what cognitive, emotional or executive function(s) that program is aimed at.

4. **Is there an independent assessment to measure my progress?** As discussed earlier, the real question is whether the improvement experienced in the program will transfer into

real life. To know if such transfer is happening we need assessments that are distinct from the exercises themselves.

5. **Is it a structured program with guidance on how many hours per week and days per week to use it?** There are no magic pills. You have to do the exercises in order to benefit, so you need clarity on the effort required.

6. **Do the exercises vary and teach me something new?** The only way to exercise your brain is by tackling novel challenges.

7. **Does the program challenge and motivate me, or does it feel like it would become easy once I learned it?** Good mental exercise requires increasing levels of difficulty and challenge.

8. **Does the program fit my personal goals?** Each individual has different goals and needs when it comes to brain health and performance. For example, some want to manage anxiety, others to improve short-term memory.

9. **Does the program fit my lifestyle?** Some interventions have shown good short-term results in lab environments, but are very intense and difficult to comply with. Others may be more appropriate for more moderate use over time.

10. **Am I ready and willing to do the program, or would it be too stressful?** Excess stress may make the whole effort counterproductive, so it is important to avoid doing things that increase your anxiety in unhealthy ways.

CHAPTER HIGHLIGHTS

- Physical exercise, balanced nutrition, stress management, and social and cognitive engagement provide a foundation for maximizing brain health and functions. Cross-training your brain builds on and goes beyond that foundation by enhancing targeted capacities.

- Each of us face different cognitive demands and have different starting points, so there is no general brain training solution for everyone and everything.

- Meditation, biofeedback, cognitive therapy and cognitive training are four types of brain training backed by scientific evidence, and emerging "conditions of use" facilitate the transfer from training to real life benefits. Technology-enabled options can make brain training more effective and accessible, if used with knowledge and with care .

INTERVIEWS

- Dr. Judith Beck – The link between brain training and weight loss.

- Dr. Martin Buschkuehl – Can intelligence be trained?

- Dr. Jerri Edwards – Improving driving skills.

- Dr. Torkel Klingberg – Expanding working memory for children with ADD/ADHD.

Interview with Dr. Judith Beck –
The link between brain training and weight loss.

BACKGROUND:

Dr. Judith Beck is the Director of the Beck Institute for Cognitive Therapy and Research and a Clinical Associate Professor of Psychology at the University of Pennsylvania. Dr. Beck is the author of *Cognitive Therapy: Basics and Beyond.* Her most recent book is *The Beck Diet Solution: Train Your Brain to Think Like a Thin Person.*

HIGHLIGHTS:

- Cognitive therapy teaches cognitive and behavioral skills to modify dysfunctional thinking and actions.

- Cognitive therapy can help dieters acquire new skills to achieve their goals.

LINKING COGNITIVE THERAPY TO WEIGHT LOSS

What is cognitive therapy?

Cognitive therapy, as developed by my father Aaron Beck, is a comprehensive system of psychotherapy, based on the idea that the way people perceive their experience influences their emotional, behavioral, and physiological responses. Part of what cognitive therapists do is to help people solve the problems they are facing today. We also teach cognitive and behavioral skills to modify dysfunctional thinking and actions.

What motivated you to bring cognitive therapy techniques to the weight-loss field by writing "The Beck Diet Solution"?

Since the beginning, I have primarily treated psychiatric outpatients with a variety of diagnoses, especially depression and anxiety. Some patients expressed weight loss as a secondary goal in treatment. I found that many of the same cognitive and behavioral techniques that helped them overcome their other problems could also help them lose weight – and keep it off.

I became particularly interested in the problem of being overweight and was able to identify specific mindsets or cognitions about food, eating, hunger, craving, perfectionism, helplessness, self-image, unfairness, deprivation, and others that needed to be targeted to help them reach their goal.

What research results back your finding that those techniques help people lose weight and keep it off?

Probably the best study published so far is the randomized controlled study by Karolinska Institute's Stahre and Hallstrom (2005). The results were striking: nearly all sixty-five patients completed the program and this short-term intervention (ten weeks, thirty hours/week) showed significant long-term weight reduction. The results were even larger, when compared to the forty individuals in the control group after eighteen months than right after the ten weeks program.

That sounds impressive. Can you explain what makes this approach so effective?

My book does not offer a diet. But it does provide tools to develop the mindset that is required for sustainable success, for modifying sabotaging thoughts and behaviors that typically follow people's initial good intentions. I help dieters acquire new skills.

So, could we say that your book is complementary to diet books?

Exactly – it helps readers set and reach their long-term goals, assuming that their diet is healthy, nutritious, and well balanced.

The main message of cognitive therapy overall, and its application in the diet world, is straightforward: problems losing weight are not a dieter's fault. Problems simply reflect lack of skills that can be acquired and mastered through practice. Dieters who read the book or workbook learn a new cognitive or behavioral skill every day for six weeks. They may practice some skills just once and incorporate others for their lifetime.

HOW TO USE COGNITIVE SKILLS
TO OVERCOME CRAVINGS

What are the cognitive and emotional skills and habits that dieters need to train?

The key ones are:

⮑ How to motivate oneself. The first task that dieters do is to write a list of the 15 of 20 reasons they want to lose weight and read that list to themselves every single day.

⮑ Planning in advance and self-monitoring behavior. A typical reason for diet failure is a strong preference for spontaneity. I ask people to prepare a plan and then I teach them the skills to stick to it.

⮑ Overcome sabotaging thoughts. Dieters have hundreds and hundreds of thoughts that lead them to engage in unhelpful eating behavior. I have dieters read cards that remind them of key points, such as: it is not worth the few moments of pleasure they will get from eating something they had not planned and that they will feel badly afterwards; that they cannot eat whatever they want, whenever they want, in whatever quantity they want, and still be thinner; that the scale is not supposed to go down every single day; and that they deserve credit for each helpful eating behavior they engage in, to name just a few.

- ⟳ Tolerate hunger and craving. Overweight people often confuse the two. You experience hunger when your stomach feels empty. Craving is an urge to eat, usually experienced in the mouth or throat, even if your stomach is full.

When do people typically experience cravings?

Triggers can be environmental (seeing or smelling food), biological (hormonal changes), social (being with others who are eating), mental (thinking about or imagining tempting food), or emotional (wanting to soothe yourself when you're upset). The trigger itself is less important than what you do about it. Dieters need to learn exactly what to say to themselves and what to do when they have cravings so they can wait until their next planned meal or snack.

How can people learn that they do not have to eat in response to hunger or craving?

I ask dieters, once they get medical clearance, to skip lunch one day and not eat between breakfast and dinner. Just doing this exercise once proves to dieters that hunger is never an emergency; that it is tolerable; that it does not keep getting worse, but instead, comes and goes; and that they do not need to "fix" their usually mild discomfort by eating.

This exercise helps dieters lose a fear of hunger. It also teaches alternative actions to help refocus attention. Feel hungry? Well, try calling a friend, taking a walk, playing a computer game, doing some email, reading a diet book, surfing the net, brushing your teeth, or doing a puzzle.

My ultimate goal is to train dieters to resist temptations by firmly saying "Eating now is not my choice," to themselves, and then naturally turning their attention back to what they had been doing or engaging in whatever activity comes next.

You said earlier that some cravings follow an emotional reaction to stressful situations. Can you elaborate on that, and explain how cognitive techniques help?

In the short term, the most effective way is to identify the problem and try to solve it. If there is nothing you can do at the moment, call a friend, do deep breathing or relaxation exercises, take a walk to clear your mind, or distract yourself in another way. Read a card that reminds you that you will certainly not be able to lose weight or keep it off if you constantly turn to food to comfort yourself when you are upset. People without weight problems generally do not turn to food when they are upset. Dieters can learn to do other things too.

And in the long term, I encourage people to examine and change their underlying beliefs and internal rules. Many people, for example, want to do everything (and expect others to do everything) in a perfect way one hundred percent of the time. That is simply impossible. This kind of thinking leads to stress.

COGNITIVE THERAPY'S IMPACT ON THE BRAIN

The title of your book includes a "train your brain" promise. Can you tell us a bit about the growing literature that analyzes the neurobiological impact of cognitive therapy?

Yes, that is a very exciting area. For years, we could only measure the impact of cognitive therapy based on psychological assessments. Today, thanks to fMRI and other neuroimaging techniques, we are starting to understand the impact our actions can have on specific parts of the brain.

For example, take spider-phobia. In a 2003 paper scientists (Paquette and colleagues) observed how, prior to the therapy, the fear induced by viewing film clips depicting spiders was correlated with significant activation of specific brain areas, like the amygdala. After the intervention was complete (one three-hour group session per week for four weeks), viewing the same spider films did not provoke activation of those areas. Those adults were able to train their brains and reduce the brain response that typically triggers automatic stress responses.

That is exactly what we find most exciting about this emerging field of neuroplasticity: the awareness that we can improve our lives by refining or "training" our brains, and the growing research behind a number of tools such as cognitive therapy.

Interview with Martin Buschkuehl –
Can intelligence be trained?

BACKGROUND:

Dr. Martin Buschkuehl is a researcher at the University of Michigan's Cognitive Neuroimaging Lab. He is one of the primary researchers involved in the cognitive training study, called "Improving Fluid Intelligence with Training of Working Memory," that has received a great deal of media attention. The study was published in April 2008 in the Proceedings of the National Academy of Sciences (PNAS). (Note: A follow-up study was published in 2011 by Drs. Susanne Jaeggi & Martin Buschkuehl showing that fluid intelligence could be trained in school-aged children as well)

HIGHLIGHTS:

- Fluid intelligence, which may be defined as the ability to deal with new problems, can be improved with training on a working memory task.

- Transfer of working memory training benefits can be observed from one task to another.

CAN INTELLIGENCE BE IMPROVED?

Could you please explain the training involved in the 2008 study published in PNAS?

We recruited 70 students around 26 years old and set half of them on a challenging computer-based cognitive training regimen, based on the so-called "n-back task." This is a very complex working memory task that involves the simultaneous presentation of visual and auditory stimuli. ("Working Memory" is the ability to hold several units of information in the mind and to manipulate them in real time.) The experimental group watched a series of screens on their computers, where a blue square appeared in various positions on a black background. Each screen appeared for half a second, with a 2.5 second gap before the next one appeared.

While this happened, the trainees also heard a series of letters that were read out at the same rate.

At first, students had to say if either the screen or the letter matched those that popped up two cycles ago. The number of cycles increased or decreased depending on how well the students performed the task. The students sat through about twenty-five minutes of training per day for either eight, twelve, seventeen, or nineteen days. They were tested on their fluid intelligence before and after the regimen using the Bochumer-Matrizen Test. The Bochumer-Matrizen Test is a problem-solving task based on the same principle as the very well known Raven's Advanced Progressive Matrices. However, it is more difficult and therefore especially suited for academic samples.

What were the results?

Participants in the experimental group did significantly better on the fluid intelligence test, which was not directly trained, than the participants in the control group. "Fluid intelligence" can be described as the ability to deal with new challenges and new problems that we encounter for the first time. Those in the control group had not gone through any training. The control group did improve slightly, but the real "trainees" outperformed them. Furthermore, we found that the improvement was dose-dependent: the more they trained, the larger the gain on fluid intelligence.

What are the particular aspects of this study that surprised you the most?

First, the clear transfer into fluid intelligence that many researchers and psychologists assume is fixed. Second, I was surprised to see that the more training, the better the outcome. The improvements did not seem to peak early.

Third, that all trained groups improved, no matter their respective starting points. In fact, students with the lowest fluid intelligence seemed to improve the most. But that was not the main focus of our study, so we cannot say much more about it.

BENEFITS OF USING COMPUTERIZED BRAIN TRAINING PROGRAMS

A common question we get about brain training software is, How are computerized programs like the one you used fundamentally different from, say, simply doing many crossword puzzles?

In terms of why our program worked, I could say that the program has some inherent properties that are, at least in this combination, unique to our training approach.

OUR PROGRAM IS:

- Fully adaptive in real-time: The person using the program is truly pushed to his or her peak level all the time, thereby "stretching" the targeted ability.

- Complex: We present a very complex task, mixing different forms of stimuli (auditory and visual) under time pressure.

- Designed for transferability: The tasks are designed in a way that does not allow for the development of task-specific "strategies" to beat the game. If one truly expands working memory capacity, this helps to ensure the transfer to non-trained tasks.

This is very different from enhancing task-specific capacities, such as memorizing lists of 100 numbers, which have been shown not to necessarily transfer to related domains.

Can you give an example of the lack of transferability of other training methods?

In Ericsson's (1998) classic paper, people who could memorize one hundred numbers using a variety of mnemonic techniques could not get even close to one hundred letters. Remembering numbers did not translate into remembering other things, so it was not a general memory capacity that had been improved.

How did participants describe the experience, and their benefits?

Many liked the training. They saw the challenge, and tried hard to push themselves through the training to see how far they could go.

We did not analyze how the fluid intelligence gains transferred into real life. But from an anecdotal point of view, many participants have shared stories of how they perceive a major benefit. Now they can follow lectures more easily, understand math better etc.

DEBATING PHYSICAL VS. MENTAL EXERCISE

There is a degree of artificial controversy these days in the media and the scientific community on the respective benefits of physical or mental exercise. What are your thoughts on the value of the different types of exercise?

We obviously need both. Physical exercise keeps the body in a good shape but especially in older people also leads to cognitive benefits. Mental exercise, like the one we used, can enhance important abilities and is most likely the most efficient way to improve a specific cognitive process but also generalizes to a broader range of skills, as we showed.

Research will need to be done to help clarify who needs what type of exercise more. Some people may get enough mental exercise through very complex jobs and what they need is physical exercise. For others, it may be the opposite.

NEXT STEPS

What are your plans now?

First, to conduct follow-up neuroimaging studies to analyze the neural basis of the improvement and second, to try to measure the benefits in real life. Our main hope is to be able to investigate and develop applications for people who need the improvement the most: children with development problems, stroke/Traumatic Brain Injury rehabilitation, and older adults.

Also, let me note that there is a cross-platform application available to train the dual n-back task and several other training tasks that we developed for other studies. Although the application is available in English, the Manual and the BrainTwister Website are not at the moment. We are about to release an English version, but unfortunately I cannot give you a release date right now. If the training program is used for research (i.e. a training study), it is provided free of charge.

Interview with Dr. Jerri Edwards – Improving driving skills.

BACKGROUND:

Dr. Jerri Edwards is an Associate Professor at University of South Florida's School of Aging Studies and Co-Investigator of the influential ACTIVE study. Dr. Edwards was trained by Dr. Karlene K. Ball, and her research is aimed at discovering how cognitive abilities can be maintained and even enhanced with advancing age.

HIGHLIGHTS:

- Speed of processing can be improved, and a significant portion of that improvement remains even after five years.

- Faster speed-of-processing seems to enable adults to react better to unexpected events that require a fast response and to reduce by 40 percent the number of dangerous maneuvers on real roads.

RESEARCH INTERESTS

Please explain to our readers your main research areas.

I am particularly interested in how cognitive interventions may help older adults to avoid or at least delay functional difficulties and thereby maintain their independence longer. Much of my work has focused on the functional ability of driving including assessing driving fitness among older adults and remediation of cognitive decline that results in driving difficulties.

Some research questions that interest me include, how can we maintain healthier lives longer? How can training improve cognitive abilities, both to improve those abilities and also to slow-down, or delay, cognitive decline? The specific cognitive ability that I have studied the most is processing speed, which is one of the cognitive skills that decline early on as we age.

RESULTS OF ACTIVE STUDY

Can you explain what cognitive processing speed is and why it is relevant to our daily lives?

Processing speed is mental quickness. Just like a computer with a 486 processor can do a lot of the same things as a computer with a Pentium 4 processor, but it takes much longer. Our minds tend to slow down with age as compared to when we were younger. We can do the same tasks; but it takes more time. Quick speed of processing is important for quick decision making in our daily lives. When you are driving, if something unexpected happens, how quickly can you notice the situation and decide how to react?

Please describe how the ACTIVE trial used the cognitive training program and what the results were found to be when they were published in the Journal of the American Medical Association in December 2006?

I was a co-investigator of the ACTIVE study, a multi-site, controlled study, with thousands of adults over sixty-five, to evaluate the effectiveness of three different cognitive training methods with three different groups:

- ⟳ The first group used a memory training program including a variety of traditional memory techniques such as mnemonics and the method of loci.

- ⟳ The second group was trained to learn inductive reasoning skills.

- ⟳ The third group was exposed to computer-based programs to train processing speed.

All three groups spent the same amount of time in their respective training programs, around two hours a week for five weeks, going through exercises of increasing difficulty. The ACTIVE study was designed to track participants' performance over a number of years. So, after this initial five week intervention, some groups received training booster sessions after one year and again after three years.

Willis and colleagues published the very positive five year results of the ACTIVE study in JAMA at the end of 2006. The most impressive result was that, when tested five years later, the participants in all three types of training had retained a significant percentage of the improvement compared to the control group. But, the results of the group that used a computer-based program to train processing speed showed more pronounced short-term and long-term improvements. Individuals who experienced improved speed of processing also showed better performance on common tasks instrumental in daily life such as quickly finding an item on a crowded pantry shelf and reading medication bottles. They also reacted to road signs more quickly. We found this transfer of training in our prior studies using the training protocol as well.

In short, significant percentages of the participants improved their memory, reasoning and information processing speed across all three methods. The most impressive result was that, when tested five years later, the participants in the computer-based program had less of a decline in the skill they were trained in than did a control group that received no cognitive training.

CLARIFYING THE CONFUSION ABOUT
THE VALUE OF BRAIN FITNESS

The results of the ACTIVE study were quite impressive and contributed in large part to the amount of media coverage about brain fitness last year. However, as you have probably seen, there s a good deal of confusion about brain fitness among the media and the public at large. Can you help our readers understand two common questions: 1) Why are new programs better than, say, doing crosswords puzzles?, and 2) Can one really say that these programs can reverse age-related decline?

To answer the first question, I would say that a crossword puzzle is not a form of cognitive training. It can be stimulating, but it is not a form of structured mental exercise that has been shown to improve specific cognitive skills – other than the skill of doing crossword puzzles, of course.

In terms of the second question, it is too early to say whether we can really reverse decline in a permanent way. There are many skills involved and the studies are not long enough to really compare different trajectories. What we can say is that by doing some exercises, one can improve cognitive speed of processing by 146-250 percent, and that a significant portion of that improvement stays even after five years. We cannot say more definitively.

But, I think it is noteworthy to be able to say that in all of the programs tested, the payoff from cognitive training, or what we can call "mental exercise," seemed far greater than we are accustomed to getting from physical exercise. Just imagine if you could say that ten hours of workouts at the gym every day this month was enough to help keep you fit five years from now.

IMPACT OF COGNITIVE TRAINING ON DRIVING A CAR

Another fascinating study that you published as a co-author in Human Factors (2003), applied a computer-based program to improving the driving-related mental skills of older adults. Can you explain that study?

Sure. Our goal was to train what is called the "useful field of view." The useful field of view is a measure of processing speed and visual attention that is critical for driving performance, and one of the areas that declines with age. It has previously been shown that this skill can be improved with training, so we wanted to see what effect it would have on the driving performance of older adults, and whether the training would be more or less effective than a traditional driving simulation course.

For the study, we divided forty-eight adults over fifty-five years old into two intervention groups of twenty-four people each. Each group received twenty hours of training. One group was exposed to a traditional driving simulator, where they learned specific driving behaviors. The other one went through the cognitive training program.

Both groups' driving performance improved right after their respective programs, but most benefits of the driving simulator disappeared by month eighteen. The speed-of-processing intervention helped participants not only improve "useful field of view," the skill that was directly trained, but it also transferred into real-life driving, and the results were sustained after eighteen months. And, by the way, the evaluation was as real as one can imagine: a fourteen mile open road evaluation. Faster speed-of-processing seemed to enable adults to react better to unexpected events that require a fast response and to reduce by forty percent the number of dangerous maneuvers on real roads (defined as those that required the training instructor to intervene during the evaluation).

LOOKING AHEAD

Research like this seems to present major opportunities for society. For example, would insurance companies, or the AARP, want to sponsor more research and evaluate whether to offer this type of training to their members? Will major employers see opportunities to improve the performance of older employees by identifying the cognitive skills that may need the most improvement and offering tailored training? We could speculate that a person with faster processing abilities will also be able to make faster decisions and learn faster. Please comment.

That makes sense, based on what we know.

Cognitive abilities evolve in different ways as we age and some typically start to decline in our thirties. Cognitive interventions may help train and improve those abilities and there is already research that strongly indicates where and how training can be useful. More research is still required to deliver more precise and tailored interventions in a variety of environments. I suspect we will see the field grow significantly – and not just for aging-related priorities. Cognitive training may become useful for a variety of health conditions, such as Parkinson's and Alzheimer's patients, for example. More research will help researchers refine assessments and training programs.

What is one recent finding or reflection, from your own work or others', that you'd like more people of all ages to know about as they try to maintain/enhance their own brain fitness?

The exercises in a brain fitness program should offer exercises that adapt to your performance. The exercises should be challenging for one to benefit. Converging evidence indicates that programs that improve divided attention skills (the ability to pay attention to two things at the same time) may be particularly important for enhancing everyday abilities among older adults.

Interview with Dr. Torkel Klingberg – Expanding working memory for children with ADD/ADHD.

BACKGROUND:

Dr. Torkel Klingberg is the Director of the Developmental Cognitive Neuroscience Lab at Karolinska Institute which is part of the Stockholm Brain Institute. Dr. Klingberg has published numerous papers in peer-reviewed publications such as the Journal of the American Academy of Child & Adolescent Psychiatry, Journal of Cognitive Neuroscience, and Nature Neuroscience on topics including the effect of working memory training itself and in combination with medication on school performance.

HIGHLIGHTS:

⮑ Working memory training can help children with attention deficits.

⮑ We may be at the beginning of a new era of computerized training with a wide range of applications.

RESEARCH ON WORKING MEMORY TRAINING

What type of research does your Developmental Cognitive Neuroscience Lab at the Karolinska Institute focus on?

The lab is addressing the questions of development and plasticity of working memory. We do that through several techniques, such as fMRI, diffusion tensor imaging to look at myelination of white matter in the brain, neural network models of working memory, and behavioral studies. In addition, I am a scientific advisor for Cogmed, the company that developed and commercializes RoboMemo.

What are the highlights of your research on the effect of working memory training?

Our paper from 2004 in Nature Neuroscience, on the effect of working memory training on brain activity, and the 2005 randomized, controlled clinical trial on the impact of working memory training specifically in kids with ADD/ADHD, have caught the most public attention.

My other research concerns the neural basis for the development and plasticity of cognitive functions during childhood, in particular the development of attention and working memory.

In short, I would say that we have shown that working memory can be improved by training and that such training helps people with attention deficits and it also improves reasoning ability overall.

What are the everyday life effects of working memory training for a child with attention deficits?

When looking at the 1,200 children who have trained in Cogmed's Stockholm Clinic, the most common effects are sustained attention, better impulse control, and improved learning ability. Parents often report that their children perform better in school and are able to keep up a coherent conversation more easily after training. Being able to hold back impulses, such as anger outbursts, and keeping better track of one's things are other everyday life benefits.

How are you making the program available?

All rights are with Cogmed, which is making this available in Sweden and started to offer this to select clinics in the US in 2006.

FUTURE OF BRAIN FITNESS PROGRAMS AND COGNITIVE TRAINING

What do you expect that we will learn over the next five years or so in the field of brain fitness programs and cognitive training?

I think that we are seeing the beginning of a new era of computerized training for a wide range of applications.

Our studies have mostly been aimed at individuals with visible problems of inattention; but, there is a wider zone concerning what you define as attention problems. We will see how Cogmed can help a larger part of the population in improving cognitive function.

What is one recent finding or reflection, from your own work or others', that you'd like more people of all ages to know about as they try to maintain/enhance their own brain fitness?

I'd like to emphasize the obvious. The key to improving both education and brain health lies in understanding how the brain works: that is where learning takes place, after all, and where we make decisions about our lifestyle and habits. For example, we need to better understand "working memory," – our ability to concentrate and to keep relevant information in our head while ignoring distractions – how people of all ages can enhance it via targeted training and aerobic exercise, and also how to protect it in stressful situations. In my new book, *The Learning Brain*, I discuss how skydivers tested just before a jump showed a 30% drop in working memory.

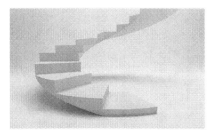

CHAPTER 9

HOW TO BE YOUR OWN BRAIN FITNESS COACH

Lifelong brain plasticity means that the way we live our live impacts, for better or for worse, our brain's structure and functioning. And, as we have emphasized throughout this guide, there is no single "magic pill" when it comes to brain fitness. Instead, there are a number of lifestyle guidelines and emerging tools that can empower you to harness your brain's neuroplasticity, helping to both maximize brain health and performance in the short-term and invest in your future by building up a cognitive reserve.

The process of putting together all the pieces of the brain fitness puzzle starts with a good understanding of how the brain and good science work (see Figure 5). From there, you can move on to addressing the lifestyle basics for good brain health: a balanced and nutritious diet, aerobic exercise, stress management, mental stimulation, and social engagement.

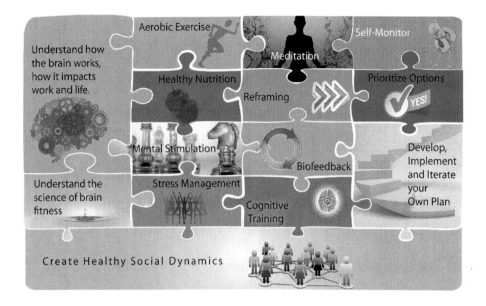

Figure 5. How to be your own brain fitness coach

Cross-training your brain can help you go further and build up capacities over time. Brain training – the structured use of methods aimed at improving specific brain functions – can be successfully performed using four main research-based methodologies: meditation, reframing, biofeedback, and cognitive training.

To truly act as your own brain fitness coach though, and make smart decisions over time, three final pieces come into play: a) prioritizing, b) self-monitoring, and c) planning.

HOW TO PRIORITIZE

Prioritizing involves establishing your personal priorities, identifying and addressing your weak points, so you can add novelty, variety and challenge to your life as necessary, and identify suitable options for action (e.g. using a biofeedback device to better regulate stress). We are providing here a few practical examples in the form of simplified vignettes that illustrate how to identify priorities based on an individual's particular starting point, needs, and goals. A summary of the person's situation is briefly presented, followed by a discussion of how that person could put together all the pieces of the brain fitness jigsaw puzzle presented above. We have ordered the examples by the age of the person in question to make it easier to track how situations and priorities tend to evolve over the lifetime.

These simplified vignettes are an effort to make the previous eight chapters come alive, and do not constitute prescriptive guidelines – our intent is to help refine your own decision-making, not to make your decisions for you. You are more than welcome to expand on and disagree with the priorities we identify.

JESSICA

Vignette: Jessica is a 16-year old girl in 11th grade. She generally eats healthy food and plays soccer twice a week. She loves spending time with her two best friends. She also spends several hours a day socializing with friends online and watching TV, which may explain her low grades in many classes this year. She's not sure what exactly she wants to do in the future, including whether to attend college or to get a job at a local retail shop run by a relative. Her parents have encouraged her to apply to college, but she is aware that attending would put a level of financial strain on the family.

Discussion: Putting in every effort to attend college is probably the best thing to do for Jessica. As discussed in Chapter 5, education is a crucial factor in brain health and fitness. It not only helps build up brain reserve but also impacts the kind of occupation, the kind of leisure activities and the kind of social relationships one is likely to have over a lifetime. As such, it is a key investment in one's brain. Having said that, Jessica needs to find the right college that engages her interests and where she will be motivated to learn, to challenge herself, and to find a stimulating job afterwards, without necessarily straining her family's resources or her future outstanding debt. Whether it is an Ivy League or a community college matters much less than whether she attends college or she doesn't.

JOHN

Vignette: John is a 25-year-old college student at a prestigious business school. He is very enthusiastic and loves to learn new concepts and strategies. Competition motivates him, although he does feel the stress and pressure. John has many friends and gets to see them often. The combination of his busy social life and his heavy work load does not give him much time to sleep or exercise, and even less time to pay attention to what he eats: pizza and a coke are at the top of the menu most days of the week.

Discussion: On top of not exercising, John obviously doesn't follow a healthy diet. Both his physical and mental performance may suffer as a result, reducing his ability to optimize his learning experience. As shown in Chapter 4, how the brain gets its fuel (glucose) impacts real-time performance: complex carbohydrates (in natural foods) provide a better, lower, and more constant intake of glucose than simple ones (in processed and sugary foods). In addition, John's lifestyle increases his risks of becoming overweight which has potential effect on cognition both in the short- and long-term. Increasing his intake of fruits and vegetables, decreasing his consumption of fast food, and doing some regular aerobic activity such as jogging, playing tennis, or hiking 2-3 times a week would probably be good steps for John to follow.

LIZ

Vignette: Liz is a 34-year-old who used to work as a librarian. She decided to stay home after her second child. She is an active participant in the parent-teacher program at school. She takes a bi-weekly aerobic class, and attends two monthly book clubs. She also finds the time to keep in touch with her good friends. Under the surface, Liz feels the pressure to be a good parent and multi-task, and sometimes has problems managing her frustration when dealing with her children or her spouse. She is not sure about what she will do after all her kids have reached school age, especially given the state of the economy.

Discussion: Liz is active physically and mentally, has a healthy diet, and a rich social life. There is one area that may become problematic: how she manages her stress. Overload, multi-tasking, and fears about the future make her sometimes slip into a depressed mood. Physical exercise helps her relieve some stress but it may not be enough. Practicing meditation could make a significant difference. She could also start using a biofeedback device to be better equipped when confronted with stressful situations and to build resilience in general.

LARRY

Vignette: Larry is a 44-year-old avid news-reader who keeps current on what is going on in his community and in the world at large. The many articles on brain health and their varied instructions for healthy behavior (Do this! Don't do that!) confuse him somewhat. He is not convinced about the effectiveness of any effort to work on one's brain fitness – the brain is what it is, especially when you are 44 years old. Still, as a naturally curious person he wants to learn more about the topic.

Discussion: Larry is outsourcing his brain to the media, which makes sense up to a point (see Chapter 2). A person can't be expected to directly read and analyze hundreds of research articles to keep current. However, in an emerging area such as brain fitness, it is important to be a well-informed and critical reader in order to make sense of new findings and/or the media coverage around those findings. He could build up his knowledge base and judgment not only by reading books like this one but also original scientific studies, which are increasingly becoming free and available online via PubMed or Google Scholar, or by visiting research labs' websites. While staying current Larry could take actions that would also help keeping his brain fit. For instance, in order to incorporate novelty, variety and challenge (as discussed in Chapter 5) and to increase meaningful social engagement (as discussed in Chapter 6), he could allocate a bit less time to passively reading newspapers and perhaps start writing a daily or weekly blog to share his main reflections and analysis with others.

HELEN

Vignette: Helen is a 48-year-old small business owner. Her job is challenging and fast-paced. Her long days at work are intellectually stimulating as they require her to solve problems, meet people, and learn new information on a regular basis. One downside of this job is the stress it creates, but Helen is usually able to manage her stress by applying principles of meditation that she learned when she was in college and has been practicing more or less consistently ever since. Helen does not always eat right (a quick sandwich here and there) but she tries to make good choices, usually preferring whole wheat bread BLT to pizza. Helen is happily married and has a few good friends with whom she likes to go out most Saturdays.

Discussion: Incorporating physical exercise in her weekly routine may be the most obvious "low-hanging fruit" for Helen and bring her several benefits. First, as discussed in Chapter 3, it may help in the short term by enhancing executive functions, which are crucial for making complex decisions and adapting to ever changing situations. Second, it may also help create a long-term neuroprotective effect so she can stay on top of her business as long as she wants to, perhaps well into her seventies. Helen could start jogging early in the morning 2-3 times a week or play racquetball games with a friend during lunch time or on the weekends.

JERRY

Vignette: Jerry is the 52 year-old CEO of a mid-sized software company. A former Marine, he considers his fitness a top priority. Currently training for an ironman competition, he maintains an intense weekly regimen that incorporates several long runs and many hours of biking and swimming, as well as strength training 3 times a week. He makes sure to eat healthy, applying the same attention to detail to his daily nutritional intake that he does for his work. He gets plenty of social contact while working, and wishes he had more time to spend with his wife and two teenage sons. His job is stressful, but he can keep the stress to a manageable level.

Discussion: Jerry is in great shape; there is no basic lifestyle area that needs major improvement. He could however take his performance to higher levels with computerized cognitive training, which he could perform during his all too frequent flights now that Internet access is common on planes. As discussed in Chapter 8, his different options would be to either choose a broad training platform or one more narrowly aimed at enhancing specific functions, such as working memory, required for superior information processing and problem-solving.

CHARLOTTE

Vignette: Charlotte is an accomplished 58-year-old reporter. She has been watching her diet and doing yoga quite intensively for years. She is noticing that it is getting harder now, especially at work, for her to concentrate and to process complex new information. She sometimes has memory lapses. Her two children no longer live with her and her husband but she is still very involved in their lives, travelling to visit them often. Charlotte is sometimes stressed by her concentration and memory problems since, as their primary caregiver, she is witnessing her own parents' physical and mental decline.

Discussion: Charlotte's busy work and family schedule does not allow her much time for herself, and when she does find that time she spends it either socializing with colleagues or at the yoga studio. Her performance problems may be due to natural age-related cognitive slowing, especially in the areas of information processing and executive attention. As shown in Chapter 8, one approach to enhance performance may be to start integrating meditation a few times a week into her schedule, perhaps reducing her overall yoga practice and combining the two. Another approach could be to try a brain training software or on-line program, maybe in the evening after a relaxing shower.

MARIO

Vignette: Mario is 61. A former elementary school teacher, he retired recently. He is enjoying retirement, finding the time at last to exercise and to see his many friends. His main problem these days is his anxiety. Especially when he can't remember other people's names. Since he saw his father go through Alzheimer's Disease, his biggest fear is to have to live through it himself, so he buys gingko biloba and other supplements in his local supermarket and does a daily cross-word puzzle.

Discussion: As outlined in Chapter 1, knowing more about his brain and how it works may be key to help Mario deal with his fears and decide when he should share these concerns with his physician. Alzheimer's disease is not necessarily hereditary: the fact that an individual's mother or father had the disease does not automatically mean that he or she will develop it also. One important risk factor is constant stress, so Mario's main priority may be to relax and take things with perspective, while simultaneously investing time in building his own cognitive reserve. Keeping in mind that memory is strongly associated with attention and anxiety may help Mario focus on what he wants to remember or eliminate distractions when he tries to learn something new. Knowledge of the brain's amazing ability to change based on experience should give Mario the confidence to start attending lifelong learning classes, perhaps taking up a new musical instrument to both release stress and stimulate his mind.

KYLE

Vignette: Kyle, a recently fully retired 67-year-old former Senior Financial Advisor, does not miss his job. He finally has the time to take care of himself, and to swim often at the local community center. Still, he does miss the constant interaction with clients and colleagues in the office. Since his wife passed away, he has not had the energy or desire to meet many people, and he is noticing a social void. He feels that his mental power and speed are not what they used to be, so he is trying to "use it or lose it" by watching documentaries on TV and by raising his daily quota of crosswords-puzzles and sudoku.

Discussion: Kyle is trying to stay cognitively engaged but, as discussed in Chapter 5, maybe not in a way that is challenging or meaningful enough. Finding opportunities to socialize and to ensure a flow of novelty, variety and challenge should probably become a stronger priority in his life. This could be achieved by volunteering or going back to work, such as taking a job providing financial planning advice to low income families for a non-profit organization. This would allow Kyle to stay socially engaged as well as keep his brain active and challenged while putting his considerable financial experience to use for a personally meaningful cause.

KELLY

Vignette: Kelly, having just celebrated her 75th birthday, has been retired for seven years now. She is in great health overall. Kelly used to love exercising, but she stopped when her mobility and strength stopped being as good as they used to. Her husband passed away 4 years ago. She has several good friends nearby but she is hesitant on the road. More and more often she prefers to stay safe at home rather than risk taking the car, and so at times she feels lonely. She worries about her memory on occasion, but generally feels good cognitively. She loves reading novels, in English as well as the half-forgotten French she learned in school.

Discussion: Kelly's brain could benefit from resuming an appropriate exercise routine, perhaps a routine of light-to-medium exercise such as walking regularly and participating in chair yoga once a week. Additionally, maintaining a stronger social network could help her stay both physically and mentally active, as she would probably feel more motivated to walk and exercise as part of a supportive group while enjoying the positive mental effects of social stimulation. She could also keep building brain reserve by joining a book club, or better yet, finding a part-time job editing the novels she so enjoys reading anyway. Given that her fear of driving seems to be stopping her from these opportunities, it may make sense for her to take safe driving classes, or even use a cognitive training software package aimed at safe driving like the one many AAA chapters have been distributing at low or no cost.

HOW TO SELF-MONITOR: BELIEFS, KNOWLEDGE, BEHAVIOR AND PERFORMANCE

In order to make appropriate decisions over time you need to self-monitor performance and behavior, as well as knowledge and beliefs. The optimal brain fitness plan will necessarily evolve over time as both the external demands and your own brain change, not to mention evolving scientific thinking.

How can this be done? We propose three separate and complementary ways:

First, to help you become more aware of your current beliefs and knowledge, we have made a list of the 55 most important brain fitness facts – in our judgment – and encourage you to read them and reflect on your level of agreement or disagreement with each of them. The list can be found in the Appendix, and follows the order of exposition in this book to make it easier to go back to the corresponding chapter if you want.

Second, to help you monitor your own behavior, we invite you to keep a brief weekly brain fitness journal in the four weeks after reading this book. Record as many much as possible that seems relevant to your brain's health: your diet, how much you exercise, your social engagements, your workload at home and at work, your daily stress levels, any memory lapses, intellectually stimulating activities, etc. At the end of the four weeks, compare your journal entries with the brain fitness jigsaw puzzle shown in Figure 5, and observe where the main gaps occur. This will give you an idea on where the "low-hanging fruit" may be waiting for you to optimize brain health and performance. And this is an iterative process, so if you find value in maintaining such a brain fitness journal over time you can simply buy a notebook or start a document on your computer or tablet and use it for this purpose.

Third, and this is perhaps the trickiest one given the limitations of the tools available today in the rapidly evolving marketplace, we encourage adventurous readers to start self-monitoring your brain performance over time using external measures of cognition, stress and resilience. How? By using some of the tools, developed by the companies identified as Market Leaders or Top Companies to Watch in SharpBrains' latest market report "Digital Brain Health Market 2012–2020: Web-based, mobile and biometrics-based technology to assess, monitor and enhance cognition and brain functioning," which are becoming available at relatively affordable prices and are user-friendly enough to provide a good experience for users willing to experiment:

- To self-monitor cognition and brain functioning overall, you could take a look at the free iPad app BrainBaseline.

- To self-monitor stress and resilience, you could take a look at the HRV biofeedback system discussed in chapter 7, EmWave Desktop.

- To self-monitor mental states such as level of concentration or excitement, you could take a look at Emotiv EPOC and NeuroSky MindWave.

Please note that, in order to reinforce the idea that we are not endorsing these products or technologies, but simply pointing out they exist for those willing to conduct their own research, we are not including product descriptions, prices or URLs.

HOW TO PLAN

We have reached the end of Part 1. You should now feel better equipped to move on to Part 2: Optimizing your own brain health and performance, by combining a comprehensive body of knowledge with a refined capability to understand and navigate options and by prioritizing what may be most relevant and beneficial to you. Assuming it took you around two weeks to read this book, please say Hello! to the many thousands of new neurons that were generated in your brain in that time. How will you take care of them? How will you take care of your brain in years to come, transforming this expanded knowledge and judgment into enlightened behaviors and actions?

We suggest a very simple plan of action:

First, identify your main weaknesses in the brain fitness jigsaw puzzle in Figure 5. Pick two pieces of the puzzle, ideally the ones with the largest disconnect between what we have discussed in this book and what you do in a typical month.

Next, select one of these to focus on first, devoting 2 hours per week to it. It would be helpful to select, by re-reading the corresponding chapter in this book, the one activity you'd like to learn more about, ideally one that you haven't been exposed to in the past and that seems aligned with your overall priorities. When you feel that this new habit is well established, move on to the second piece of the puzzle that you pick and follow the same procedure.

Finally, share your journey with other people to enhance your learning and motivation, as well as to help others by passing on your newfound knowledge. You could do so in person, via social media via your own blog.

To conclude, let us end this guide with the same words we used to open it:

We dedicate this book to your Unique Brain, and your Unique Mind.

AFTERWORD

As you go through life, your brain undergoes extraordinary development. Your brain is the most adaptable, modifiable organ in your body, and it can change both positively and negatively by how you use it each day. Just by reading this book, your brain has been changed.

How has your brain been altered throughout your life? How may it change in years and decades ahead? The good news is that much of the age-related decline is likely avoidable and even reversible. The fact that you bought and have read this book to the very end tells me you are motivated to do something about your brain performance. Our cognitive brain health tends to decline over time because we let it, but you can be your own brain health fitness coach to maximize brain function. Growing brain research shows that a majority of individuals can make their brain smarter every single day.

When I first met Alvaro after having spoken at the impressive 2012 SharpBrains Virtual Summit, our brains connected as we shared our thoughts on what major gaps needed to be filled to achieve greater brain gains for individual and global brain health. As a cognitive brain scientist, my life has been dedicated to discovering ways to optimize brain health and applying rapidly emerging innovations to make a difference in people's lives. Alvaro and I come together from disparate disciplines, but we both see brain performance as the most vital and urgent frontier to build a healthier, more economically productive society.

It typically takes twenty to forty years or more for scientific discoveries to meaningfully benefit human life. We cannot wait that long.

It would be too late for the majority of people today. None of us can afford to let our brains decline – not even for a day. You would not accept that for your heart, eyes, or lungs, so why allow such slippage for your most valued asset? Increasing research and scientific discoveries from my research center, the Center for BrainHealth at The University of Texas at Dallas, and others have shown that everyone can increase their intellectual capital, maximize their cognitive potential, and harness the immense capacity of their brain to rewire itself in health, and even after brain injury or brain disease.

How can we extend the brain span to more closely match the extensive gains in the human lifespan?

As I offer reflections on the brain health advice and scientific evidence unfolded throughout this book, I hope you begin to think differently about your brain and actively embrace the exciting and promising reality that your brain's health is the cause of the century. I challenge you to:

- Update any outdated beliefs about the brain.

- Sort out and stop habits that are impairing your brain performance.

- Spend time on meaningful real-life activities that demand vital decision-making and complex problem solving.

- Begin today preparing a plan for next week. What is one tangible step you are willing to take to better your brain health?

- Become a vocal ambassador of brain health to all those around you — whether at work, home, community or play.

You have taken an important first step to becoming an active member of the Brain Fitness Movement by reading this book. You are never too young or too old to commit to adopting beneficial brain health habits that challenge and enhance your brain's capacity to think and act smarter. And keep in mind that…

Your health starts and ends with your brain's health.

Your brain is the most vital organ and supports everyday things you do, including your ability to think, learn, reason, create, problem solve, imagine, decide, or plan. You should start and end every day thinking about how well you have tended to the health of your brain, whatever life stage you are in. It is just as essential to measure, monitor and maximize your brain fitness as it is to measure, monitor and maximize your physical fitness. In fact, more can be done to keep your brain healthy than any other part of your body.

As a start to your new commitment to brain health, take seriously the recommendations and ideas generated from reading *The Sharp-Brains Guide to Brain Fitness*. I invite you to impact, imagine, innovate, and inspire.

- **Impact.** We always want something easy to do, like a certain number of puzzles to complete each day or a magic pill to take, to make us think smarter and keep our brain healthy. But simplistic formulas do not have a substantial and lasting impact on such a complex organ as our brain.

- **Imagine.** We know more about the universe than we do about the human brain, but brain science is a fast growing field of exploration. Scientific research shows every individual builds a unique brain by how they use their brain every day. You control your brain's destiny. Imagine the limitless possibilities.

- **Innovate.** Today, scientists and innovators worldwide are taking advantage of innovative and sophisticated technological advances to document and measure dramatic, rapid rewiring at all levels of the brain – from brain blood flow, to synapses, and even to entire brain networks. Design and innovate your own brain workouts to take advantage of all these brain gains.

- **Inspire.** Inspire others around you to adopt brain habits and encourage them to become involved in complex cognitive activities. Become a role model and show how to reduce high levels of stress, engage in proper nutrition, and retain rich social engagements.

In the past ten years brain scientists have discovered much more about how the brain works, how to improve brain health and performance over time, and how doing so contributes to overall health and well-being. Join us in making sure your best brain years are ahead of you. **Without brain health, you do not have health.**

Sandra Bond Chapman, PhD

Founder and Chief Director – Center for BrainHealth
Dee Wyly Distinguished University Professor
The University of Texas at Dallas
Author, Make Your Brain Smarter (Free Press, 2013)

APPENDIX

55 IMPORTANT BRAIN FITNESS FACTS

Top 3 Brain Facts

1. There is not only one "It" in "Use It or Lose It." The brain is composed of a number of specialized units. Our life and productivity depend on a variety of brain functions, not just one.

2. Genes do not determine the fate of our brains. Lifelong neuroplasticity allows our lifestyles and actions to play a meaningful role in how our brains physically evolve, especially given longer life expectancy.

3. Aging does not mean automatic decline. There is nothing inherently fixed in the precise trajectory of how our brain functions evolve as we age.

Top 7 Smart News Reader Facts

1. Just because a study is everywhere in the media does not necessarily mean it is a sound and relevant study.

2. Randomized controlled trials (RCT) provide the most compelling evidence that a treatment or intervention causes an effect on human behavior. They are more powerful than observational studies.

3. The 2010 extensive meta-analysis by the NIH is a great starting point to understand what factors may benefit brain functions: It reports a fairly consistent and protective effect of cognitive engagement, physical exercise, and the Mediterranean diet on cognitive functions.

4. In the 2010 SharpBrains survey that included 1,910 self-selected respondents aged 20 to 60+, the ability to manage stressful situations, the concentration power to avoid distractions, and being able to recognize and manage one's emotions emerged as the most important brain functions to thrive personally and professionally.

5. The priority for brain optimization does not have to be prevention of dementia.

6. We all have cognitive biases that may influence our decisions (e.g., the tendency to overvalue events or results that are recent compared to older ones).

7. We will not have a Magic Pill or General Solution to solve all our cognitive challenges any time soon. A multi-pronged approach is recommended, centered around nutrition, stress management, and both physical and mental exercise.

Top 4 Brain and Physical Exercise Facts

1. Physical exercise has been shown to enhance brain physiology in animals and, more recently, in humans.

2. Physical exercise improves learning and other brain functions through increased brain volume, blood supply and growth hormone levels in the body.

3. Of all the types of physical exercise, cardiovascular exercise that gets the heart beating – from walking to skiing, tennis and basketball – has been shown to have the greatest effect.

4. Aerobic exercise for at least thirty to sixty minutes per day, three days a week, seems to be the best regimen.

Top 11 Brain and Nutrition Facts

1. The brain needs a lot of energy: It extracts approximately 50% of the oxygen and 10% of the glucose from arterial blood.

2. The blood-brain barrier (BBB) prevents some substances in the blood (such as bacteria) from entering the brain while allowing the diffusion of oxygen and glucose towards it.

3. Intake of omega-3 fatty acids is associated with decreased risk of cognitive decline.

4. Intake of vegetables (and thus antioxidants) is associated with decreased risks of cognitive decline and dementia.

5. Tobacco use increases risks of cognitive decline and dementia.

6. Moderate doses of caffeine can increase alertness but there is no clear sustained lifetime benefit.

7. Light-to-moderate alcohol consumption lowers the risk of dementia.

8. Diabetes increases the risk of cognitive decline and dementia.

9. Obesity is associated with cognitive deficits, but the nature of the relationship is not clear.

10. Taking vitamins B6, B12, E, C, and beta carotene does not boost cognitive function and does not affect the risks of cognitive decline or dementia

11. There is strong evidence that Gingko Biloba does not reduce risk of developing dementia. It doesn't seem to enhance brain function either.

Top 8 Mental Challenge Facts

1. Mental stimulation strengthens the connections between neurons (synapses), thus improving neuron survival and cognitive functioning.

2. Mental stimulation also helps build cognitive reserve, helping the brain be better protected against potential pathology.

3. Routine activities do not challenge the brain. Keeping up the challenge requires going to the next level of difficulty or trying something new.

4. Reading, writing, playing board or card games, doing crosswords and other puzzles, and participating in organized group discussions can be cognitively challenging activities.

5. Musical training increases brain reserve and is neuroprotective.

6. As is speaking several languages.

7. The only leisure activity that has been associated with reduced cognitive function is watching television.

8. A good way to increase variety and learning is to try new activities, including some at which you are not good at (if you like to sing, try painting or dancing).

Top 6 Brain and Social Engagement Facts

1. Higher social engagement is associated with higher cognitive functioning and reduced risks of cognitive decline.

2. The larger and the more complex a person's social network is, the bigger his or her's amygdala (a brain structure that plays a major role in our emotional responses).

3. Volunteering helps lower mortality and depression rates, and slows down rates of decline in physical health and cognitive function.

4. Larger social network sizes are associated with better cognitive function.

5. Belonging to a social group combines the benefits of social engagement with those triggered by the activity performed by the group.

6. A dance club will combine benefits from social and physical

stimulation, while a book club will combine intellectual and social engagement.

Top 6 Brain and Stress Facts

1. Chronic stress reduces and can even inhibit neurogenesis.
2. Memory and general mental flexibility are impaired by chronic stress.
3. Aerobic exercise helps counteract the effects of stress on the brain as it leads to the creation of new neurons and connections in the brain.
4. Relaxation lowers blood pressure and slows respiration and metabolism, decreasing the physiological symptoms of stress.
5. Social relationships and humor can be used to fight stress.
6. Meditation and biofeedback devices that measure heart rate variability are the two research-based tools that have been clearly shown to successfully teach one to control physiological stress responses and thereby increase long-term emotional regulation.

Top 10 Brain Training Facts

1. Medication is not the only or even main hope for cognitive enhancement. Non-invasive interventions can have comparable and more durable effects, side effect-free.
2. Not all brain activities or exercises are equal. Varied and targeted exercises are the necessary ingredients in brain training so that a wide range of brain functions can be stimulated.
3. Brain training can work assuming some key conditions are met.
4. "Brain age" is a fiction: No two individuals have the same brain or cognitive functioning. Consequently, brain training cannot be said to roll back "brain age" by 10, 20, or 30 years.

5. Not all individuals share the same brain fitness priorities. As with physical fitness, people must ask themselves: What functions do I need to improve? In what timeframe?

6. Brain training is more effortful, and its effects are more specific, compared to a challenging leisure activity.

7. Since brain training aims at enhancing a specific function or functions, one must determine which functions need training in order to select the type of methodology that will work.

8. Defined as the structured use of cognitive exercises or techniques aimed at improving specific brain functions, brain training includes a range of research-supported methodologies: meditation, cognitive therapy, and cognitive training (via computerized programs).

9. Meditation can train one's emotional control and attentional focus. Eight weeks of a Mindfulness Based Stress Reduction (MBSR) program can be enough to increase brain volume in areas involved in learning, memory and emotion regulation.

10. Cognitive training software programs vary widely. Some provide an overall brain workout while others target specific functions or abilities (i.e., driving, or working memory).

ABOUT SHARPBRAINS

SharpBrains is an independent market research firm tracking health and productivity applications of cognitive and affective neuroscience, with special emphasis on non-invasive technology and the growing needs of an aging population.

Our mission is to provide organizations and individuals with independent, research-based information and guidance that is up-to-date and actionable. We offer access to the latest insights and best practices for those who want to be at the forefront of the application of neuroscience knowledge. To that end, we publish a biannual state-of-the market report series and produce an annual global and virtual professional conference, as well as publish resources such as this book to educate and empower everyone with a brain.

A key informational resource is our website and blog, www.SharpBrains.com, which attracts 100,000+ monthly readers and 50,000+ eNewsletter subscribers with a variety of resources, including:

- A blog maintained by SharpBrains staff and experts and updated several times per week

- A searchable archive of hundreds of past articles

- A free monthly eNewsletter

- A number of helpful lists, questions & answers and brain teasers

ABOUT THE AUTHORS

Alvaro Fernandez, co-author

Alvaro Fernandez is the Chief Executive Officer of SharpBrains, a leading market research firm and innovation think tank in the emerging field of brain fitness. He is a nationally-known speaker and expert, quoted by The New York Times, The Wall Street Journal, New Scientist, CNN, and other media outlets. Alvaro has an MBA and MA in Education from Stanford University, and a BA in Economics from Universidad de Deusto. He started his career at McKinsey & Company and led the launch and turnaround of several publishing and education companies in the US and Europe. In March 2012 Alvaro was named a Young Global Leader by the World Economic Forum (WEF), an honor which recognizes the most distinguished young leaders under the age of 40 from around the world.

Elkhonon Goldberg, co-author

Elkhonon Goldberg, Ph.D., is SharpBrains' Chief Scientific Adviser. He is an author, scientist, educator and clinician, internationally renowned for his clinical work, research, writing and teaching in neuropsychology and cognitive neuroscience. Dr. Goldberg is a Clinical Professor, Department of Neurology at New York University School of Medicine, and Diplomate of The American Board of Professional Psychology in Clinical Neuropsychology. A student and close associate of the great neuropsychologist Alexander Luria, Dr. Goldberg has continued to advance Luria's scientific and clinical tradition, and written popular science books such as *The Executive Brain: Frontal Lobes and The Civilized Mind, The Wisdom Paradox: How Your Mind Can Grow Stronger As Your Brain Grows Older*, and *The New Executive Brain: Frontal Lobes in a Complex World*.

Pascale Michelon, contributing author

Pascale Michelon, Ph.D. in Cognitive Psychology, is a scientist, educator and writer. Dr. Michelon started her career as a Research Scientist at Washington University in Saint Louis where she conducted behavioral and neuroimaging studies to better understand how the brain processes and memorizes visual information. She published many peer-reviewed articles and received awards for her scientific work. She is now an Adjunct Faculty at Washington University and facilitates memory workshops in the St. Louis area. She was the Research Manager for the first Edition of the SharpBrains Guide to Brain Fitness, and recently wrote *Max Your Memory*, an illustrated memory workbook.

ACKNOWLEDGEMENTS

This book was not written by a few individuals working in a vacuum. Over a hundred great minds contributed directly or indirectly by shaping the ideas we discussed, helping condense and synthesize the extended body of relevant scientific research, and providing new perspectives and insights.

In particular, we would like to acknowledge the meaningful contributions of the hundreds of participants in the three annual SharpBrains Virtual Summits so far – specifically to the Speakers and Moderators who kindly donated their valuable time and insight:

- Dr. Tracy Packiam Alloway PhD, Assistant Professor at the University of North Florida

- Dr. Daphne Bavelier, Professor at the Department of Brain and Cognitive Sciences at the University of Rochester

- Dr. Gregory Bayer, CEO of Brain Resource

- Sharon Begley, Senior Health & Science Correspondent at Reuters

- Dr. Robert Bilder, Chief of Medical Psychology-Neuropsychology at the UCLA Semel Institute for Neuroscience

- Shlomo Breznitz, President of CogniFit

- Nolan Bushnell, Founder of Atari

- Tim Chang, Managing Director at Mayfield Fund

- Dr. Sandra Bond Chapman, Founder and Director of the Center for BrainHealth at the University of Texas at Dallas

- Peter Christianson, President of Young Drivers of Canada
- Michael Cole, CEO of Vivity Labs
- David Coleiro, Partner at Strategic North
- Prof. Cary Cooper, Science Co-ordination Chair at the Foresight Project on Mental Capital and Wellbeing
- Dr. Brenda Dann-Messier, Assistant Secretary for Vocational and Adult Education at the US Department of Education
- Dr. David Darby, Chief Medical Officer at CogState
- Marian C. Diamond, PhD, Professor of Neuroscience and Anatomy at UC-Berkeley
- Dr. P Murali Doraiswamy, Biological Psychiatry Division Head at Duke University
- Kristi Durazo, Senior Strategy Advisor at the American Heart Association
- Dr. Jerri Edwards, Associate Professor at the University of South Florida
- Keith Epstein, Senior Strategic Advisor at AARP
- Dr. Martha Farah, Director of the Center for Neuroscience and Society at the University of Pennsylvania
- Dr. Sheryl Flynn, CEO of Blue Marble Game Co
- Lindsay Gaskins, CEO of Marbles: The Brain Store
- Dr. Adam Gazzaley, Director of the Neuroscience Imaging Center at the University of California, San Francisco
- Ken Gibson, President of LearningRx
- Prof. James Giordano, Director of the Center for Neurotechnology Studies and Vice President for Academic Programs at the Potomac Institute for Policy Studies
- Annette Goodman, Chief Education Officer at the Arrowsmith Program
- Dr. Evian Gordon, Executive Chairman of Brain Resource

- Eric B. Gordon, CEO of Atentiv
- Dr. C. Shawn Green, Assistant Professor at the University of Wisconsin-Madison
- Dr. Walter Greenleaf, CEO of Virtually Better
- Muki Hansteen-Izora, Senior Design Researcher and Strategist at Intel's Digital Group
- Dr. Joe Hardy, VP of Research and Development at Lumos Labs
- Kathleen Herath, Associate Vice President Health & Productivity at Nationwide Insurance
- Dr. Laurence Hirshberg, Director of the NeuroDevelopment Center
- Charles (Chuck) House, Executive Director of Media X
- Jonas Jendi, former CEO of Cogmed
- Dr. Charles Jennings, Director of the McGovern Institute Neuro-technology Program at MIT
- Dr. Holly Jimison, Associate Professor at the Department of Medical Informatics & Clinical Epidemiology, Oregon Health & Science University
- Dr. Jeffrey Kaye, Director of ORCATECH
- Dr. Dharma Singh Khalsa, President of the Alzheimer's Research and Prevention Foundation
- Peter Kissinger, President of the AAA Foundation for Traffic Safety
- Robin Klaus, Chairman and CEO of Club One
- D. Torkel Klinberg, Professor of Cognitive Science at the Karolinska Institute
- Dr. Kenneth Kosik, Co-Director of the UC Santa Barbara Neuroscience Research Institute
- Corinna E. Lathan, Founder and CEO of AnthroTronix
- Tan Le, CEO of Emotiv Lifesciences
- Richard Levinson, President of Attention Control Systems

- Veronika Litinski, Director of the MaRS Venture Group
- Dr. Stephen Macknik, Director of the Laboratory of Behavioral Neurophysiology at the Barrow Neurological Institute
- Dr. Henry Mahncke, CEO of Posit Science
- Dr. Michael Merzenich, Emeritus Professor at UCSF
- Dan Michel, CEO of Dakim
- Alexandra Morehouse, VP Brand Management at Kaiser Permanente
- Margaret Morris, Senior Researcher at Intel's Digital Health Group
- Brian Mossop, Community Editor at Wired
- Michel Noir, CEO of SBT / HappyNeuron
- Dr. Alvaro Pascual-Leone, Director of the Berenson-Allen Center for Non-Invasive Brain Stimulation at Harvard Medical School
- Dr. Misha Pavel, Biomedical Engineering Division Head at Oregon Health & Science University and Program Director for the National Science Foundation's Smart Health and Wellbeing Program
- Lena Perelman, Director of Community Outreach at SCAN Health Plan
- Dr. Michael Posner, Professor Emeritus at the University of Oregon
- Paula Psyllakis, Senior Policy Advisor at the Ontario Ministry of Research and Innovation
- Patty Purpur, Director of the Stanford Health Promotion Network
- Dr. William Reichman, President of Baycrest
- Dr. Peter Reiner, Co-Founder of the National Core for Neuroethics at the University of British Columbia
- Dr. John Reppas, Director of Public Policy for the Neurotechnology Industry Organization
- Dr. Albert "Skip"Rizzo, Co-Director VR Psych Lab at USC
- Beverly Sanborn, Vice President of Activities and Memory Programs at Belmont Village Senior Living

- Kunal Sarkar, CEO of Lumos Labs
- Lisa Schoonerman, Co-Founder of vibrantBrains
- Dr. Gary Small, Director of the Center on Aging at the UCLA Semel Institute for Neuroscience & Human Behavior
- Nigel Smith, Strategy and Innovation Director at the AARP
- Dr. Joshua Steinerman, Assistant Professor at Albert Einstein College of Medicine – Montefiore Medical Center
- Dr. Yaakov Stern, Cognitive Neuroscience Division Leader at Columbia University
- Rodney Stoops, Vice President at Providence Place Retirement Community
- Kate Sullivan, Director of the Brain Fitness Center at Walter Reed National Military Medical Center
- Dr. Michael Valenzuela, Leader of the Regenerative Neuroscience Group at UNSW
- Dr. Sophia Vinogradov, Interim Vice Chair of Department of Psychiatry at UCSF
- Dr. Molly Wagster, Chief of the Behavioral and Systems Neuroscience Branch in the Division of Neuroscience at the National Institute on Aging (NIA)
- Thomas M. Warden, Vice President of Allstate's Research and Planning Center (ARPC)
- Mark Watson, Director of Community Outreach at the Eaton Educational Group
- Dr. Keith Wesnes, Practice Leader at United BioSource Corporation
- David Whitehouse, Chief Medical Officer of OptumHealth Behavioral Solutions
- Dr. Peter Whitehouse, Professor of Neurology at Case Western Reserve University

- Dr. Jesse Wright, Director of the Depression Center at the University of Louisville
- Stanley Yang, CEO of NeuroSky
- Dr. Elizabeth Zelinski, Professor at the USC David School of Gerontology

GLOSSARY

ACTIVE Study: The largest properly randomized and controlled trial ever published in the area of brain training. Participants, who were in their 70's, were exposed to different forms of mental training: reasoning, memory and speed training. They showed an improvement in the skills trained and retained a significant percentage of this improvement when tested five years later.

Aerobic Exercise: see Physical Exercise

Amygdala: A part of the limbic system, located deep inside the temporal lobe of the brain. It plays a major role in processing and memorizing emotions, especially fear.

Attention: The ability to sustain concentration on a particular object, action or thought; to manage competing demands in our environment. Supported primarily by networks in the parietal and frontal lobes, it includes focused attention and divided attention.

"BBC Brain Training Study": Refers to a study published in 2010 and sponsored by the BBC (British Broadcasting Corporation). Touted as evidence that brain training doesn't work, it was criticized by scientists on a number of grounds.

Beta-Amyloid: The protein that constitutes the main component of the amyloid plaques found in the brains of individuals suffering from Alzheimer's disease.

Biofeedback: Biofeedback hardware devices measure and graphically display various physiological variables such as skin conductivity and heart rate variability, so that users can learn to self-adjust.

Blood-Brain Barrier (BBB): A barrier surrounding the brain that prevents some materials from entering while allowing others in (e.g., glucose), thereby helping to maintain a constant environment for the brain.

Brain Fitness: The general state of feeling alert, in control, productive. Having the mental abilities required to function in society, in our occupations, and in our communities.

Brain Functions: See Cognitive Abilities

Brain Reserve: See Cognitive Reserve

Brain Training (or Cognitive Training): Refers to the structured use of methodologies designed to build targeted brain-based networks and capacities. Its aim is to improve specific brain functions. It encompasses computerized brain fitness products but also research-based methodologies such as meditation.

Cognitive Abilities (or Brain functions): Brain-based skills we need to carry out any task. They have more to do with the mechanisms of how we learn, remember, and pay attention rather than with any actual knowledge. Examples are memory, attention, and language skills.

Cognitive Bias: Reliable tendencies toward specific judgment errors, that result from peculiarities of our mental processing systems.

Cognitive Decline: Deterioration in cognitive function. Age-related cognitive decline is a normal process characterized mainly by increasing difficulties in learning and speed of information processing.

Cognitive Engagement/Stimulation: Refers to the lifelong participation in activities that are challenging for the brain and may thus trigger neuroplastic changes.

Cognitive Reserve (or Brain Reserve): Theory that addresses the fact that individuals vary considerably in the severity of cognitive aging and clinical dementia. Mental stimulation, education and occupational level are believed to be major active components of building a cognitive reserve that can help resist the effects of brain disease on cognition.

Cognitive Therapy (CT): Type of therapy based on the idea that the way people perceive their experience influences their behaviors and emotions. The therapist teaches the patient cognitive and behavioral skills to modify his or her dysfunctional thinking and actions. CT aims at improving specific cognitive skills or behaviors (such as planning and mental flexibility), as well as at helping the individual combat the symptoms and undesirable effects of clinical conditions (such as depression, obsessive-compulsive disorders, or phobias).

Cognitive Training: see Brain Training

Computerized Brain Training Software Program: Fully-automated applications designed to assess and enhance cognitive abilities. Adaptive software-based programs present the user with various tools to exercise different brain structures and cognitive skills by continually responding to performance and increasing difficulty level incrementally. These software products can be delivered either online or via software.

Emotion: Complex states that involve both a physiological, or bodily, experience and a psychological, or cognitive, experience. They are closely related to motivation.

Emotional Resilience: The ability to adapt to stressful situations or crises. It entails emotional awareness and a sense of control over one's emotions.

Executive Functions: Abilities that enable goal-oriented behavior, such as the ability to plan, and execute a goal. They include mental flexibility, theory of mind, anticipation, self-regulation, working memory and inhibition.

Glial Cell: A category of cells found in the brain. They are even more numerous than neurons, and help neurons function normally.

Glucose: A form of sugar, it is the brain's source of fuel. Glucose in the blood comes mostly from carbohydrates.

Heart Rate Variability (HRV): Refers to the beat-to-beat alterations in heart rate (the time interval between heart beats).

Hebb's Rule: Refers to the principle that brain cells that fire together, wire together. Neurons that are often active at the same time tend to become associated and end up connecting one to another.

Hippocampus: A part of the limbic system, located deep inside the temporal lobe. Plays a major role in memory formation and spatial navigation.

Hypothalamus: A part of the limbic system, the hypothalamus helps control things like body temperature, hunger, and sleep, primarily through the release of hormones.

IMPACT Study: A randomized controlled trial involving over 500 participants that tested the efficiency of the software developed by Posit Science to train auditory processing.

Language and Auditory Processing: Skills allowing us to differentiate and comprehend sounds and generate verbal output. They are supported by the temporal, parietal, and frontal lobes.

Limbic System: A group of several structures (including the amygdala, the hippocampus, and the hypothalamus) that collaborate to process emotions, regulate memories, produce hormones, and manage sexual arousal and circadian rhythms.

Meditation: A collection of techniques that share the ultimate goal of going beyond one's automatic thinking and being to get into a "deeper," or more grounded state. It can help build up the control of attention of emotional arousal.

Mediterranean Diet: Typically involves high intakes of vegetables, fruits, cereals and unsaturated fats (mostly in the form of olive oil), low intakes of dairy products, meat and saturated fats, moderate intake of fish and a regular but moderate alcohol consumption.

Meta-Analysis: A statistical method that combines the results of several studies addressing the same hypotheses. It enables the assessment of the size and generalizability of an effect.

Mild Cognitive Impairment (MCI): A transitional stage between normal aging and dementia of Alzheimer's (AD) or other types. Some people with MCI eventually develop dementia and others do not.

Motor Skills: The ability to mobilize our muscles and bodies or manipulate objects, either automatically or voluntarily.

Neocortex: The outer layer of each hemisphere, which controls a variety of higher mental functions, such as perceptual processing, attention, and decision making. Can be divided into four distinct areas: the occipital, temporal, parietal, and frontal lobes.

Neurofeedback: A type of biofeedback relying on electrophysiological measures of brain activity.

Neurogenesis: The process by which neurons continue to be born throughout our lives.

Neuroimaging: Techniques that either directly or indirectly image the structure, function, or physiology of the brain. Recent techniques (such as fMRI) have enabled researchers to understand better the living human brain.

Neuroplasticity: The brain's ability to reorganize itself throughout life.

Nerve Growth Factors: A family of substances produced by the body to help maintain and repair neurons. An example is Brain-Derived Neurotrophic Factor (BDNF), a protein that helps support the functioning of existing neurons in the brain and encourages the growth of new neurons and synapses.

NIH Meta-Analysis (2010): A comprehensive and systematic meta-analysis commissioned by the U.S. National Institute of Health (NIH), in which the authors analyzed the results of 25 reviews of studies and 250 single studies to understand which factors are associated with reduction of risks of AD and cognitive decline.

Observational Study: A research study in which the researchers only observe associations (or correlations) between different factors. Causation cannot be inferred from such a study.

Omega-3 fatty acids: An important part of any nutritious diet (along with omega-6 fatty acids), and a brain-healthy diet in particular. Can be found in cold-water fish, kiwi, and some nuts.

Parasympathetic Nervous System (PNS): The system responsible for managing the "rest-and-digest" activities that occur when the body is at rest, such as salivation, urination, sexual arousal, and digestion.

Physical Exercise: The effortful activity of particular parts of our bodies. It includes aerobic exercise (generally light-to-moderate in intensity, longer in duration) and anaerobic exercise (generally high in intensity, shorter in duration), which depend on different energy sources.

PubMed: A very useful tool to search for published studies. PubMed is a service of the U.S. National Library of Medicine that includes over 16 million citations from MEDLINE and other life science journals for biomedical articles back to the 1950s. It includes links to full text articles and other related resources.

Randomized Controlled Trial (RCT): A research study in which participants are randomly assigned to a test and a control/placebo groups. A RCT provides the most compelling evidence that the treatment or intervention tested has a causal effect on human health or behavior.

Stress: Stress is a common emotion triggered by an experience or situation in which the demands on an organism exceed its natural capacity to regulate itself. When the stress is ongoing and long-term, it is referred to as chronic stress, and can interfere with neural function and negatively impact the immune system's defenses.

Sympathetic Nervous System (SNS): The system responsible for managing the "fight-or-flight" responses. Its functions range from constricting blood vessels, activating sweat glands, and dilating pupils, to increasing heart rate and its force of contraction.

Synapse: Specialized connections by which neurons exchange chemical information, in the form of neurotransmitters. Each neuron can have up to 10,000 synapses with other neurons.

Synaptogenesis: The formation of new connections (synapses between neurons). It is a type of neuroplasticity.

Transfer: The translation of training effects to untrained tasks and to benefits in everyday life.

Video Game: An electronic game that requires the user to interact with a platform such as a computer or a console. Its purpose is entertainment and not cognitive improvement.

(Higher-Order) Visual and Spatial Processing: The ability to process incoming visual information and visualize images and scenarios, and the ability to process spatial relationships between objects.

Working Memory: The ability to keep information current for a short period while using this information. Working memory is used for controlling attention, and deficits in working memory capacity lead to attention problems.

REFERENCES

CHAPTER 1

Damasio, A. (1995). Descartes' error: Emotion, reason, and the human brain. Penguin Press.

De Beaumont L, Theoret H, Mongeon D at al. (2009). Brain function decline in healthy retired athletes who sustained their last sports concussion in early adulthood. Brain, 132(3), 695-708.

Draganski, B., Gaser, C., Kempermann, G., Kuhn, H. G., Winkler, J., Buchel, C., & May A. (2006). Temporal and spatial dynamics of brain structure changes during extensive learning. The Journal of Neuroscience, 261231, 6314-6317.

Gardner, H. (1983). Frames of Mind: The theory of multiple intelligences. New York: Basic Books.

Gaser, C. & Schlaug, G. (2003). Brain structures differ between musicians and non-musicians. The Journal of Neuroscience, 23, 9240-9245.

Grossmann, I., Na, J., Varnum, M. E. W., Park, De. D., Kitayama, S., & Nisbett, R. E. (2010). Reasoning about social conflicts improves into old age. PNAS, 107, 7246–7250.

Guskiewicz, K. M., Marshall, S. W., Bailes, J., McCrea, M., Cantu, R. C., Randolph, C., & Jordan, B. D. (2005). Association between recurrent concussion and late-life cognitive impairment in retired professional football players. Neurosurgery, 57(4),719-26

Kolb, D. (1983). Experiential learning: Experience as the source of learning and development. FT Press.

Maguire, E. A., Woollett, K., & Spiers, H. J. (2006). London taxi drivers and bus drivers: A structural MRI and neuropsychological analysis. Hippocampus, 16, 1091-1101.

Mechelli, A., Crinion, J. T., Noppeney, U. , O'Doherty, J., Ashburner, J., Frackowiak, R. S., & Price, C. J. (2004). Structural plasticity in the bilingual brain. Nature, 431, 757.

Rueda, M. R., Posner, M. I., & Rothbart, M. K. (2005) The development of executive attention: contributions to the emergence of self-regulation. Developmental Neuropsychology, 28, 573-594.

Rueda, M. R., Rothbart, M. K.., Saccamanno, L., & Posner, M. I. (2005) Training, maturation and genetic influences on the development of executive attention. Proceedings of the National Academy of Sciences, 102, 14931-14936.

Singh-Manoux, A., Kivimaki, M., Glymour, M. M., Elbaz, A., Berr, C., Ebmeier, K. P., Ferrie, J. E., & Dugravot, A. (2012). Timing of onset of cognitive decline: results from Whitehall II prospective cohort study. BMJ, 344, 1-8.

Sylwester, R. (2007). The adolescent brain: Reaching for autonomy. Corwin Press.

Sylwester, R. (2010). A Child's Brain: The Need for Nurture. Corwin Press.

Tang, Y., Ma, Y., Wang, J., Fan, Y., Feng, S., Lu, Q., et al. (2007). Short-term meditation training improves attention and self-regulation. Proceedings of the National Academy of Sciences, 104(43), 17152-17156.

Williams, J. W., Plassman, B. L., Burke, J., Holsinger, T., & Benjamin, S. (2010). Preventing Alzheimer's Disease and Cognitive Decline. NIH Evidence Report: AHRQ Publication.

Woodruff, L., & Woodruff, B. (2007). In an instant: A Family's journey of love and healing. Random House.

Woollett, K. & Maguire, E. A. (2011). Acquiring "the Knowledge" of London's Layout Drives Structural Brain Changes. Current Biology, 21(24), 2109-2114.

Zull, J. E. (2002). The Art of changing the brain: Enriching the practice of teaching by exploring the biology of learning. Stylus Publishing: Sterling, VA.

CHAPTER 2

Hölzel, B. K., Carmody, J., Vangel, M., Congleton, C., Yerramsetti, S. M., Gard, T., & Lazar, S. W. (2011). Mindfulness practice leads to increases in regional brain gray matter density. Psychiatry Research: Neuroimaging, 191 (1), 36-43.

Luders, E., Kurth, F., Mayer, E. A., Toga, A. W., Narr, K. L., & Gaser, C. (2012). The Unique Brain Anatomy of Meditation Practitioners: Alterations in Cortical Gyrification. *Frontiers in Human Neuroscience*, 2012; 6 DOI: 10.3389/fnhum.2012.00034

Lutz, A., Greischar, L. L., Rawlings, N. B., Ricard, M., & Davidson, R. J. (2004). Long-term meditators self-induce high-amplitude gamma synchrony during mental practice. *PNAS*, 101(46), 16369-16373.

Owen, A. M., Hampshire, A., Grahn, J. A., Stenton, R., Dajani, S., Burns, A. S., et al., (2010). Putting brain training to the test. Nature, 465(7299), 775-778.

Pascual-Leone, A., Amedi, A., Fregni, F., & Merabet, L. B. (2005). The Plastic Human Brain Cortex. Annu. Rev. Neurosci., 28, 377–401.

Fox, M. D., Halko, M. A., Eldaief, M. C., & Pascual-Leone, A. (2012) Measuring and manipulating brain connectivity with resting state functional connectivity magnetic resonance imaging (fcMRI) and transcranial magnetic stimulation (TMS). Neuroimage, Mar 19. [Epub ahead of print].

Prochaska, J. O., Norcross, J. C., & DiClemente, C. C. (1994). Changing for good: The revolutionary program that explains the six stages of change and teaches you how to free yourself from bad habits. New York: W. Morrow.

Tang, Y., Lu, Q., Geng, X., Stein, E.A., Yang, Y., & Posner, M.I. (2010) Short term mental training induces white-matter changes in the anterior cingulate PNAS 107 16649-16652

Tang, Y-Y.,Lu, Q., Fan, M., Yang, Y., & Posner,M.I. (2012) Mechanisms of White Matter Changes Induced by Meditation Proceedings of the National Academy of Sciences USA 109 (26) 10570-10574 doi10/.1073pnas.1207817109

Williams, J. W., Plassman, B. L., Burke, J., Holsinger, T., & Benjamin, S. (2010). Preventing Alzheimer's Disease and Cognitive Decline. NIH Evidence Report: AHRQ Publication.

CHAPTER 3

Angevaren, M., Aufdemkampe, G., Verhaar, H. J. J., et al. (2008). Physical activity and enhanced fitness to improve cognitive function in older people without known cognitive impairment. Cochrane Database of Systematic Reviews, (3):CD005381.

Basak, C., Boot, W.R., Voss, M.W., & Kramer, A.F. (2008). Can Training in a Real-Time Strategy Videogame Attenuate Cognitive Decline in Older Adults? Psychology & Aging, 23(4), 765-777.

Chaddock, L., Erickson, K., Prakash, R., Kim, J.S., Voss, M., VanPatter, M., Pontifex, M., Raine, L., Konkel, A., Hillman, C. Cohen, N. & Kramer, A.F. (2010a). A neuroimaging investigation of the association between aerobic fitness, hippocampal volume, and memory performance in preadolescent children. Brain Research, 1358, 172-83.

Chaddock, L., Erickson, K., Prakash, R., VanPatter, M., Voss, M., Pontifex, M., Raine, L., Hillman, C. & Kramer, A. F. (2010b). Basal ganglia volume is associated with aerobic fitness in preadolescent children. Developmental Neuroscience, 32, 249-256.

Colcombe, S. J., Erickson, K. I., Scalf, P. E., Kim, J. S., Prakash, R., McAuley, E., Elavsky, S., Marquez, D. X., Hu, L., & Kramer, A. F. (2006). Aerobic exercise training increases brain volume in aging humans. Journal of Gerontology, 61A(11), 1166–1170.

Colcombe, S., & Kramer, A. F. (2003). Fitness effects on the cognitive function of older adults: A Meta-Analytic study. Psychological Science, 14 (2), 125-130.

Davis, J. C., Marra, C. A., Beattie, B. L., Robertson, M. C., Najafzadeh, M., Graf, P., Nagamatsu, L. S., & Liu-Ambrose, T. (2010). Sustained Cognitive and Economic Benefits of Resistance Training Among Community- Dwelling Senior Women: A 1-Year Follow-up Study of the Brain Power Study. Arch Intern Med., 170(22), 2036-2038.

Eriksson, P. S., Perfilieva, E., Bjork-Eriksson, T., Alborn, A. N., Norborg, C., Peterson, D., & Gage, F. H. (1998). Neurogenesis in the adult human hippocampus. Nature Medicine, 4(11): 1313-1317, 1998.

Erickson, K. I., Raji, C.A., Lopez, O.L., Becker, J.T., Rosano, C., Newman, A.B., Gach, H.M., Thompson, P.M., Ho, A.J. & Kuller, L. H. (2010). Physical activity predicts gray matter volume in late adulthood: The Cardiovascular Health Study. Neurology, 75, 1415.

Erickson, K. I., Ruchika, K. I., Prakash, S., Voss, M. W., Chaddock, L., Hu, L., Morris, K. S., White, S. M., Wójcicki, T. R., McAuley, E., & Kramer, A. F. (2009). Aerobic fitness is associated with hippocampal volume in elderly humans. Hippocampus, 19(10), 1030-1039.

Faherty, C. J., Shepherd, K. R., Herasimtschuk, A., & Smeyne, R. J. (2005). Environmental enrichment in adulthood eliminates neuronal death in experimental Parkinsonism. Molecular Brain Research, 134(1), 170-179.

Flöel, A., Ruscheweyh, R., Krüger, K., Willeme, C., Winter, B., Völker, K., Lohmann, H., Zitzmann, M., Mooren, F., Breitenstein, C., & Knecht, S. (2010). Physical activity and memory functions: Are neurotrophins and cerebral gray matter volume the missing link? NeuroImage, 49, 2756–2763.

Gage, F. H., Kempermann, G., & Song, H. (2007). Adult Neurogenesis. Cold Spring Harbor Laboratory Press, NY.

Geda, Y. E., Roberts, R. O., Knopman, D. S., Christianson, T. J., Pankratz, V. S., Ivnik, R. J., Boeve, B. F., Tangalos, E. G., Petersen, R. C., & Rocca, W. A. (2010) Physical exercise, aging, and mild cognitive impairment: a population-based study. Arch Neurol., 67(1). 80-6.

Griffin, E. W., Mullally, S., Foley, C., Warmington, S. A., O'Mara, S. M., & Kelly, A. M. (2011). Aerobic exercise improves hippocampal function and increases BDNF in the serum of young adult males. Physiol Behav., 104(5), 934-41.

Lautenschlager, N. T., Cox, K. L., Flicker, L., et al. (2008). Effect of physical activity on cognitive function in older adults at risk for Alzheimer disease: a randomized trial. JAMA, 300(9),1027-37. Nagamatsu, L. S., et al (2012). Resistance training promotes cognitive and functional brain plasticity in seniors with probable mild cognitive impairment. Arch Intern Med, 172(8), 666-668.

Nunes, A., & Kramer, A.F. (2009). Experience-based mitigation of age-related performance declines: Evidence from air traffic control. Journal of Experimental Psychology: Applied, 15(1), 12-24.

Scarmeas, N., Luchsinger, J., Schupf, N., Brickman, A., Cosentino, S., Tang M., & Stern, Y. (2009). Physical activity, diet, and risk of Alzheimer disease. JAMA, 302, 627-637.

Williams, J. W., Plassman, B. L., Burke, J., Holsinger, T., & Benjamin, S. (2010). Preventing Alzheimer's Disease and Cognitive Decline. NIH Evidence Report: AHRQ Publication.

CHAPTER 4

DeKosky, S. T., et al. (2008). Ginkgo biloba for prevention of dementia: a randomized controlled trial. Journal of the American Medical Association, 300, 2253-2262.

Féart, C., Samieri, C., Rondeau, V., Amieva, H., Portet, F., Dartigues, J.-F., Scarmeas, N., & Barberger-Gateau, P. (2009), Adherence to a Mediterranean *diet*, *cognitive decline*, and risk of dementia. Journal of the American Medical Association, 302(6), 638-648.

Fitzpatrick, A. L., Kuller, L. H., Lopez, O.L., et al. (2009). Midlife and late-life obesity and the risk of dementia: cardiovascular health study. Arch Neurol., 66(3), 336-342.

Gagnon C., Greenwood C.E. & Bherer L. 2010. The acute effects of glucose ingestion on attentional control in fasting healthy older adults. *Psychopharmacology, 211 (3)*, 337-346.

Johnson-Kozlow, M., Kritz-Silverstein, D., Barrett-Connor, E., & Morton, D. (2002). Coffee consumption and cognitive function among older adults. American Journal Of Epidemiology, 156 (9), 842-850.

Kaye, J. (2009). Ginkgo biloba prevention trials: More than an ounce of prevention learned. Archives of Neurology, 66(5), 652-654.

Laitala, V. S., Kaprio, J., Koskenvuo, M., Räihä, I., Rinne, J. O., & Silventoinen, K. (2009). Coffee drinking in middle age is not associated with cognitive performance in old age. The American Journal Of Clinical Nutrition, 90 (3), 640-646.

Lindsay, J., Laurin, D., Verreault, R., Hébert, R., Helliwell, B., Hill, G. B., & McDowell, I. (2002). Risk factors for Alzheimer's disease: a prospective analysis from the Canadian Study of Health and Aging. American Journal Of Epidemiology, 156 (5), 445-453.

McCleary, L. (2007). The Brain Trust Program: A scientifically based three-part plan to improve memory, elevate mood, enhance attention, alleviate migraine and menopausal symptoms, and boost mental energy. Perigee Trade.

Piscitelli, S. C, Burstein, A. H., Chaitt, D., Alfaro, R. M., Falloon, J. (2001). Indinavir concentrations and St John's wort. Lancet, 357, 1210.

Scarmeas, N., Luchsinger, J. A., Schupf, N., Brickman, A. M., Cosentino, S., Tang, M. X., & Stern, Y. (2009). Physical activity, diet, and risk of Alzheimer disease. Journal of the American Medical Association, 302(6), 627-637.

Scarmeas, N., Stern, Y., Mayeux, R., Manly, J. J., Schupf, N., & Luchsinger, J. A. (2009). Mediterranean Diet and Mild Cognitive Impairment. *Arch Neurol.*, *66*(2), 216-225.

Smith, E., Hay, P., Campbell, L., & Trollor, J. N. (2011). A review of the association between obesity and cognitive function across the lifespan: implications for novel approaches to prevention and treatment. Obesity Reviews, 12(9), 740–755.

Snitz, B. E., et al. (2009). Ginkgo biloba for preventing cognitive decline in older adults: A randomized trial. Journal of the American Medical Association, 302(24), 2663-2670.

Strachan, M. W. J., Price, J. F., & Frier, B. M. (2008). Diabetes, cognitive impairment, and dementia. BMJ, 336(7634), 6.

Sofi, F., Macchi, C., Abbate, R., Gensini, G. F., & Casini, A. (2010). Effectiveness of the Mediterranean diet: Can it help delay or prevent Alzheimer's disease? Journal of Alzheimer's Disease, 20(3), 795-801.

van Boxtel, M. P. J., Schmitt, J. A. J., Bosma, H., Jolles, J. (2003). The effects of habitual caffeine use on cognitive change: a longitudinal perspective. Pharmacology, Biochemistry and Behavior, 75(4), 921-927.

Williams, J. W., Plassman, B. L., Burke, J., Holsinger, T., & Benjamin, S. (2010). Preventing Alzheimer's Disease and Cognitive Decline. NIH Evidence Report: AHRQ Publication.

CHAPTER 5

American Society on Aging (2006). ASA-Metlife Foundation Attitudes and Awareness of Brain Health Poll.

Basak, C., Boot, W. R., Voss, M. W., & Kramer, A. G. (2008). Can training in a real-time strategy video game attenuate cognitive decline in older adults? Psychology and Aging, 23(4), 765-777

Bialystok, E., Fergus I.M. Craik, F. I. M., & Freedman, M. (2007). Bilingualism as a protection against the onset of symptoms of dementia. Neuropsychologi, 45, 459–464.

Dehaene, S., Pegado, F, Braga, L. W., Ventura, P. Filho, G. N., Jobert, A., Dehaene-Lambertz, G., Kolinsky, R., Morais, J., & Cohen, L. (2010). How Learning to Read Changes the Cortical Networks for Vision and Language. Science, 330 (6009), 1359-1364.

Garbin, G., Sanjuan, A., Forn, C., Bustamante, J. C., Rodriguez-Pujadas, A., Belloch, V., Hernandez, M., Costa, A., & Ávila. C. (2010). Bridging language and attention: Brain basis of the impact of bilingualism on cognitive control. NeuroImage, 53, 1272-1278.

Gopher, D., Weil, M., & Bareket, T. (1994). Transfer of skill from a computer game trainer to flight. Human Factors, 36, 1-19.

Green, C.S. & Bavelier, D. (2007). Action video game experience alters the spatial resolution of vision. Psychological Science, 18(1), 88–94.

Green, C. S., Pouget, A., & Bavelier, D. (2010). Improved Probabilistic Inference as a General Learning Mechanism with Action Video Games. Current Biology, 20(17), 1573-1579.

Greitemeyer, T., & Osswald, S. (2010). Effects of prosocial video games on prosocial behavior. Journal of Personality and Social Psychology, 98 (2), 211-221.

Hanna-Pladdy, B., & MacKay, A. (2011). The Relation Between Instrumental Musical Activity and Cognitive Aging. Neuropsychology, 25 (3), 378-86.

Hambrick, D. Z., Sathouse, T. A., & Meinz, E. J. (1999). Predictors of crossword puzzle proficiency and moderators of age-cognition relations. Journal of Experimental Psychology: General, 128, 131-164.

Katzman, R., Aronson, M., Fuld, P., Kawas, C., Brown, T., Morgenstern, H., Frishman, W., Gidez, L., Eder, H., & Ooi, W.L. (1989). Development of dementing illnesses in an 80-year-old volunteer cohort. Annals of Neurology, 25, 317-324.

Kraus, N., & Chandrasekaran, B. (2010). Music training for the development of auditory skills. Nature Reviews Neuroscience, 11, 599-605.

Landau, S. M., & D'Esposito, M. (2006). Sequence learning in pianists and non-pianists: An fMRI study of motor expertise. Cognitive, Journal Affective, & Behavioral Neuroscience, 6 (3), 246-259.

Landau, S. M. et al. (2012). Association of Lifetime Cognitive Engagement and Low Beta-Amyloid Deposition. Arch Neurol. Published online January 23, 2012. doi:10.1001/archneurol.2011.2748

Li, R., Polat, U., Makous, W. & Bavelier, D. (2009). Enhancing the contrast sensitivity function through action video game playing. Nature Neuroscience, 12(5), 527–8.

McDougall, S. & House, B. (2012). Brain training in older adults: Evidence of transfer to memory span performance and pseudo-Matthew effects. Aging, Neuropsychology, and Cognition, 19 (1–2), 195–221.

Nouchi, R., Taki, Y., Takeuchi, H., Hashizume, H., Akitsuki, Y., Shigemune, Y., Sekiguchi, A., Kotozaki, Y., Tsukiura,T., Yomogida, Y., & Kawashima, R. (2012). Brain Training Game Improves Executive Functions and Processing Speed in the Elderly: A Randomized Controlled Trial. PLoS ONE 7(1): e29676.

Rohwedder, S., and Willis., R. J. (2010). Mental Retirement. Journal of Economic Perspectives, 24(1), 119–38.

Scarmeas, N., Levy, G., Tang, M. X., Manly, J., & Stern, Y. (2001). Influence of leisure activity on the incidence of Alzheimer's disease. Neurology, 57, 2236-2242.

Schooler, C., Mulatu, M. S., & Oates, G. (1999). The continuing effects of substantially complex work on the intellectual functioning of older workers. Psychology and Aging, 14, 483-506.

Snowdon, D. A., Ostwald, S. K., Kane, R. L., & Keenan, N. L. (1989). Years of life with good and poor mental and physical function in the elderly. Journal of Clinical Epidemiology, 42, 1055-1066.

Stern, Y. (2002). What is cognitive reserve? Theory and research application of the reserve concept. Journal of Int. Neuropsych. Soc., 8, 448-460.

Wang, J.Y., Zhou, D.H., Li, J., Zhang, M., Deng, J., Tang, M., et al. (2006). Leisure activity and risk of cognitive impairment: The Chongqing aging study. Neurology, 66(6), 911–913.

Williams, J. W., Plassman, B. L., Burke, J., Holsinger, T., & Benjamin, S. (2010). Preventing Alzheimer's Disease and Cognitive Decline. NIH Evidence Report: AHRQ Publication.

Wilson, R. H., Barnes, L. L., Aggarwal, N. T., Boyle, P. A., Hebert, L. E., Mendes de Leon, C. F., & Evanc, D. A. (2010). Cognitive activity and the cognitive morbidity of Alzheimer's disease. Neurology, 75, 990–996.

Wilson, R.S., Bennett, D.A., Bienias, J.L., Aggarwal, N.T., Mendes de Leon, C.F., Morris, M.C., Schneider, J. A., & Evans, D. A. (2002). Cognitive activity and incident AD in a population-based sample of older persons. Neurology, 59, 1910-1914.

Yaffe, K., Weston, A., Graff-Radford, N. R., Satterfield, S., Simonsick, E. M., Younkin, S. G., Younkin, L. H., Kuller, L., Ayonayon, H. N., Ding, J., & Harris, T. B. (2011). Association of Plasma β-Amyloid Level and Cognitive Reserve With Subsequent Cognitive Decline. JAMA, 305(3), 261-266.

Zelinski, E. M., & Burnight, K. P. (1997). Sixteen-year longitudinal and time lag changes in memory and cognition in older adults. Psychology and Aging, 12(3), 503-513.

Zelinski et al. (on-going). The IMPACT Study: A randomized controlled trial of a brain plasticity-based training program for age-related decline.

CHAPTER 6

Bickart, K. C., Wright, C. I., Dautoff, R. J., Dickerson, B. C., & Feldman Barrett, L. (2011). Amygdala volume and social network size in humans. Nature Neuroscience, 14, 163–164.

Bennett, D.A., Schneider, J.A., Tang, Y., Arnold, S.E., & Wilson, R.S. (2006). The effect of social networks on the relation between Alzheimer's disease pathology and level of cognitive function in old people: A longitudinal cohort study. Lancet Neurology, 5(5), 406– 412.

Bowling, A., & Grundy, E. (1998). The association between social networks and mortality in later life. Rev. Clin. Gerontology, 8, 353–61.

Carlson, M. C., Erickson, K. I., Kramer, A. F., Voss, M. W., Bolea, N., Mielke, M., et al. (2009). Evidence for neurocognitive plasticity in at-risk older adults: The Experience Corps program. Journals of Gerontology Series A: Biological Sciences and Medical Sciences, 64(12), 1275–1282.

Conroy, R. M., Golden, J., Jeffaresa, I., O'Neill, D., & McGee, H. (2010). Boredom-proneness, loneliness, social engagement and depression and their association with cognitive function in older people: A population study. Psychology, Health & Medicine,15(4), 463-473.

Diamond, A., Barnett, W. S., Thomas, J., and Munro, S. (2007). Preschool program improves cognitive control. *Science* 318, 1387–1388.

Dunbar, R. I. M. (1992) Neocortex Size As A Constraint On Group Size In Primates. J. Human Evo, 22, 469.

Dunbar, R. I. M. et al. (in press). Journal of Computer-Mediated Communication.

Fratiglioni, L., Paillard-Borg, S., & Winblad, B. (2004). An active and socially integrated lifestyle in late life might protect against dementia. Lancet Neurology, 3(6), 343–353.

Goncalves, B., Perra, N., & Vespignani, A. (2011). Modeling Users' Activity on Twitter Networks: Validation of Dunbar's Number. PLoS ONE 6(8): e22656.

Harris, A. H., & Thoresen, C. E. (2005). Volunteering is associated with delayed mortality in older people: Analysis of the longitudinal study of aging. Journal of Health Psychology, 10(6), 739–752.

Hsu, H. C. (2007). Does social participation by the elderly reduce mortality and cognitive impairment? Aging & Mental Health, 11(6), 699-707.

Jackson, J. J., Hill, P. L., Payne, B. R., Roberts, B. W., & Stine-Morrow, E. A. L. (2012, Jan 16). Can an old dog learn (and want to experience) new tricks? Cognitive training increases openness to experience in older adults. Psychology and Aging, Advance online pub.

Krueger, K. R., Wilson, R. S., Kamenetsky, J. M., Barnes, L. L., Bienias, J. L., & Bennett, D. A. (2009). Social engagement and cognitive function in old age. Experimental Aging Research, 35(1), 45-60.

Morrow-Howell, N., Hinterlong, J., Rozario, P. A., & Tang, F. (2003). Effects of volunteering on the well-being of older adults. Journals of Gerontology, Series B: Psychological Sciences and Social Sciences, 58(3), S137–145.

Pollet, T. V., Roberts, S. G. B., & Dunbar, R. I. M. (2011). Use of Social Network Sites and Instant Messaging Does Not Lead to Increased Offline Social Network Size, or to Emotionally Closer Relationships with Offline Network Members. Cyberpsychology, Behavior, and Social Networking, 14(4), 253-258.

Reis, H. T., Smith, S. M., Carmichael, C. L., Caprariello, P. A., Tsai, F. F., Rodrigues, A., & Maniaci, M. R. (2010). Are you happy for me? How sharing positive events with others provides personal and interpersonal benefits. Journal of Personality and Social Psychology, 99(2), 311-329.

Saczynski, J. S., Pfeifer, L. A., Masaki, K., Korf, E. S., Laurin, D., White, L., & Launer, L. J. (2006). The effect of social engagement on incident dementia: The Honolulu-Asia Aging Study. American Journal of Epidemiology, 163(5), 433–440.

Williams, J. W., Plassman, B. L., Burke, J., Holsinger, T., & Benjamin, S. (2010). Preventing Alzheimer's Disease and Cognitive Decline. NIH Evidence Report: AHRQ Publication

Ybarra, O., Burnstein, E., Winkielman, P., Keller, M. C., Manis, M., Chan, E., & Rodriguez, J. (2008). Mental exercising through simple socializing: Social interaction promotes general cognitive functioning. Personality and Social Psychology Bulletin, 34, 248-259.

Ybarra, O., Winkielman, P. Yeh, I., Burnstein, E., & Kavanagh, L. (2011). Friends (and sometimes enemies) with cognitive benefits: Which types of social interactions boost executive functioning? Social Psychological and Personality Science, 2, 253-261.

CHAPTER 7

Berk., L. S., Tan, S. A., Fry, W. F., Napier, B. J., Lee, J. W., Hubbard, R. W., Lewis, J. E., & Eby, W. C. (1989). Neuroendocrine and stress hormone changes during mirthful laughter. Am J Med Sci., 298(6), 390-396.

Berman, M. G., Jonides, J., & Kaplan, S. (2008). The Cognitive Benefits of Interacting With Nature. Psychological Science, 19(12), 1207-1212.

Bennett, M. P., Zeller, J. M., Rosenberg, L., & McCann J. (2002). The effect of mirthful laughter on stress and natural killer cell activity. Altern Ther Health Med., 9(2), 38-45.

Cowen, P. J. (2002). Hypercortisolism cortisol, serotonin and depression: all stressed out? The British Journal of Psychiatry, 180, 99-100.

Elliott, W., Izzo, J., White, W. B., Rosing, D., Snyder, C. S., Alter, A., Gavish, B., & Black, H. R. (2004). Graded Blood Pressure Reduction in Hypertensive Outpatients Associated with Use of a Device to Assist with Slow Breathing. J Clin Hypertens, 6(10), 553-559.

Emmons, R. A. (2007). Thanks: How the New Science of Gratitude Can Make You Happier. Boston: Houghton Mifflin.

Emmons, R. A. & McCullough, M. E. (2003). Counting Blessings versus Burdens: An Experimental Investigation of Gratitude and Subjective Well-Being in Daily Life. Journal of Personality and Social Psychology, 84(2), 377–389.

Gordon, N. S. (2003). The neural basis of joy and sadness: A functional magnetic resonance imaging study of the neuro-affective effects of music, laughter and crying. ProQuest Information & Learning, 64, 997.

Grossman, E., Grossman, A., Schein, M. H., Zimlichman, R., & Gavish, B. (2001). Breathing-control lowers blood pressure. Journal of Human Hypertension, 15, 263-269.

Head, D., Singh, T., & Bugg, J. M. (2012). The moderating role of exercise on stress-related effects on the hippocampus and memory in later adulthood. Neuropsychology, (Jan 30, ahead of print)

Hofmann, S. G., Sawyer, A. T., Witt, A. A., & Oh, D. (2010). The effect of mindfulness-based therapy on anxiety and depression: A meta-analytic review. J Consult Clin Psychol. 78(2),169-83.

Hölzel, B. K., Carmody, J., Evans, K. C., Hoge, E. A., Dusek, J. A., Morgan, L., et al (2010). Stress reduction correlates with structural changes in the amygdala. Social, Cognitive, and Affective Neuroscience, 5 (1): 11-17.

Jamieson, J. P., Mendes, W. B., Blackstock, E., & Schmader, T. (2010). Turning the knots in your stomach into bows: Reappraising arousal improves performance on the GRE. Journal of Experimental Social Psychology, 46, 208–212.

Lemaire, J. B., Wallace, J. E., Lewin, A. M., de Grood, J., & Schaefer, J. P. (2011). The Effect of a Biofeedback-based Stress Management Tool on Physician Stress: A Randomized Controlled Clinical Trial. Open Medicine, 5(4), E154.

Lupien, S. J., Fiocco, A., Wan, N., Maheu, F., Lord, C., Schramek, T., & Tu, M. T. (2005). Stress hormones and human memory function across the lifespan. Psychoneuroendocrinology, 30(3), 225-242.

McCraty, R., Atkinson, M., Arguelles, L., & Lipsenthal, L. (2009). New Hope for Correctional Officers: An Innovative Program for Reducing Stress and Health Risks. Appl Psych and Biofeedback, 34(4), 251-272.

Miller, G. (2011). Social neuroscience. Why loneliness is hazardous to your health. Science, 14, 331(6014), 138-40.

Newberg, A., D'Aquili, E., & Rause, V. (2001). Why God won't go away: Brain science and the biology of belief. Ballantine Books.

Newberg, A. & Waldman, M. R. (2006). Why we believe what we believe: Uncovering our biological need for meaning, spirituality, and truth. Free Press.

Newberg, A., & Waldman, M. (2009). How God Changes the Brain: Breakthrough Findings from a Leading Neuroscientist. Ballantine Books.

Nyklicek, I., & Kuijpers, K. F. (2008). Effects of mindfulness-based stress reduction intervention on psychological well-being and quality of life: Is increased mindfulness indeed the mechanism? Annals of Behavioral Medicine, 35(3), 331–340.

Pines, E. W., Rauschhuber, M. L., Norgan, G. H., Cook, J. D., Canchola, L., Richardson, C., & Jones, M. E. (2011). Stress resiliency, psychological empowerment and conflict management styles among baccalaureate nursing students. J. Adv. Nurs (Epub ahead of print)

Prinsloo, GE, Rauch, HGL, Lambert, MI, Muench, F, Noakes, TD & Derman WE (2010). The Effect of Short Duration Heart Rate Variability (HRV) Biofeedback on Cognitive Performance During Laboratory Induced Cognitive Stress. Published online in Wiley Online Library (wileyonlinelibrary.com) DOI: 10.1002/acp.1750

Sapolsky, R. M. (2004). Why zebras don't get ulcers. Owl Books.

Schein, M., Gavish, B., Herz, M., Rosner-Kahana, D., Naveh, P., Knishkowy, B., Zlotnikov, E., Ben-Zvi, N., & Melmed, R. N. (2001). Treating hypertension with a device that slows and regularizes breathing: A randomised, double-blind controlled study. Journal of Human Hypertension, 15, 271-278.

Segrin, C., & Passalacqua, S. A. (2010). Functions of loneliness, social support, health behaviors, and stress in association with poor health. Health Commun., 25, 312-22.

Sherlin, L., Gevirtz, R., Wyckoff, S., & Muench, F. (2009). Effects of Respiratory Sinus Arrhythmia Biofeedback Versus Passive Biofeedback Control, International Journal of Stress Management, 16(3), 233-248.

Steenbarger, B, N. (2006). Enhancing Trader Performance: Proven Strategies From the Cutting Edge of Trading Psychology. Wiley.

Steenbarger, B. N. (2003). The Psychology of Trading: Tools and Techniques for Minding the Markets. Wiley.

Williams, J. W., Plassman, B. L., Burke, J., Holsinger, T., & Benjamin, S. (2010). Preventing Alzheimer's Disease and Cognitive Decline. NIH Evidence Report: AHRQ Publication

Zeidan, F., Johnson, S. K., Diamond, B. J., David, Z., Paula Goolkasian, P. (2010). Mindfulness meditation improves cognition: Evidence of brief mental training. Consciousness and Cognition, 19, 597–605.

CHAPTER 8

Ball, K., Edwards, J. D., Ross, L. A., McGwin, G. (2010). Cognitive Training Decreases Motor Vehicle Collision Involvement of Older Drivers. Journal of the American Geriatrics Society, 58(11), 2107–2113.

Barnes, D. E., Yaffe, K., Belfor, N., Jagust, W. J., DeCarli, C., Reed, B. R., & Kramer, J. H. (2009). Computer-Based Cognitive Training for Mild Cognitive Impairment: Results from a Pilot Randomized, Controlled Trial. Alzheimer Dis Assoc Disord. 2009 Jul–Sep; 23(3): 205–210.

Beck, A. (1979). Cognitive therapy and the emotional disorders. Plume.

Beck, J. S. (1995). Cognitive Therapy: Basics and Beyond. Guilford Press.

Beck, J. S. (2007). The Beck diet solution: Train your brain to think like a thin person. Oxmoor House.

Beck, S. J., Hanson, C. A., Puffenberger, S. S., Benningerb, K. L., & Benninger, W. B. (2010). A Controlled Trial of Working Memory Training for Children and Adolescents with ADHD. Journal of Clinical Child & Adolescent Psychology, 39(6), 825-836.

Berry, A. S., Zanto, T. P., Clapp, W. C., Hardy, J. L., Delahunt, P. B., Mahncke, H. W., & Gazzaley, A. (2010). The Influence of Perceptual Training on Working Memory in Older Adults. PLoS One, 5(7): e11537.

Brehmer, Y., Rieckmann, A., Bellander, M., Westerberg, H., Fischer, H., & Bäckman, L. (2011). Neural correlates of training-related working-memory gains in old age. Neurolmgae, 58(4), 1110-1120.

Davidson, R. J., Kabat-Zinn, J., Schumacher, J., Rosenkranz, M., Muller, D., Santorelli, S. F., Urbanowski, F., Harrington, A., Bonus, K. and Sheridan, J. F. (2003). Alterations in brain and immune function produced by mindfulness meditation. Psychosomatic Medicine, 65, 564-570.

Edwards, J. D., … & Mahncke, H. W. (2009). Cognitive speed of processing training delays driving cessation. The Journals of Gerontology: Series A: Biological Sciences and Medical Sciences, 64A(12), 1262-1267.

Finn, M., & McDonald, S. (2012). Computerised Cognitive Training for Older Persons With Mild Cognitive Impairment: A Pilot Study Using a Randomised Controlled Trial Design. Brain Impairment, 12(3), 187-199.

Hofmann, S. G., Sawyer, A. T., Witt, A. A., & Oh, D. (2010). The effect of mindfulness-based therapy on anxiety and depression: A meta-analytic review. J Consult Clin Psychol. 78(2),169-83.

Hölzel, B. K., Carmody, J., Vangel, M., Congleton, C., Yerramsetti, S. M., Gard, T., & Lazar, S. W. (2011). Mindfulness practice leads to increases in regional brain gray matter density. Psychiatry Research: Neuroimaging, 191 (1), 36-43.

Jackson, J. J., Hill, P. L., Payne, B. R., Roberts, B. W., & Stine-Morrow, E. A. L. (2012). Can an old dog learn (and want to experience) new tricks? Cognitive training increases openness to experience in older adults. Psychology and Aging, Advance online pub.

Jaeggi, S. M., Buschkuehl, M., Jonides, J., & Perrig, W. J. (2008). Improving fluid intelligence with training on working memory. Proceedings of the National Academy of Sciences of the United States of America, 105(19), 6829-6833.

Jaeggi, S. M., Buschkuehl, M., Jonides, J., & Shah, P. (2011). Short- and long-term benefits of cognitive training. PNAS, 108 (25), 10081-10086.

Jobe, J. B., Smith, D. M., Ball, K., Tennstedt, S. L., Marsiske, M., Willis, S. L., Rebok, G. W., Morris, J. N., Helmers, K. F., Leveck, M. D., Kleinman, K. (2001). ACTIVE: A cognitive intervention trail to promote independence in older adults. Control Clinical Trials, 22(4), 453-479.

Klingberg, T., Fernell, E., Olesen, P. J., Johnson, M., Gustafsson, P., Dahlström, K., Gillberg, C. G., Forssberg, H., & Westerberg, H. (2005). Computerized training of working memory in children with ADHD-A randomized, controlled trial. J. American Academy of Child and Adolescent Psychiatry, 44(2), 177-186.

Lundqvist, A., Grundström, K., Samuelsson, K., & Rönnberg, J. (2010). Computerized training of working memory in a group of patients suffering from acquired brain injury. Brain Inj., 24(10),1173-83.

MacLean, K. A., Ferrer, E., …& Saron, C. (2010). Intensive meditation training improves perceptual discrimination and sustained attention. Psychological Science, 21(6), 829-839.

Mahncke, H. W., Connor, B. B., Appelman, J., Ahsanuddin, O. N., Hardy, J. L., Wood, R. A., Joyce, N. M., Boniske, T., Atkins, S. M., & Merzenich, M. M. (2006). Memory enhancement in healthy older adults using a brain plasticity-based training program: A randomized, controlled study. PNAS, 103(33), 12523-12528.

Moore, A., & Malinowski, P. (2009). Meditation, mindfulness and cognitive flexibility. Consciousness and Cognition, 18(1), 176–186.

Paquette, V., Levesque, J., Mensour, B., Leroux, J. M., Beaudoin, G., Bourgouin, P., et al. (2003). Effects of cognitive-behavioral therapy on the neural correlates of spider phobia. Neuroimage, 18, 401-409.

Peretz, C., Korczyn, A. D., Shatil, E., Aharonson, V., Birnboim, S., & Giladi, N. (2012). Computer-based, personalized cognitive training versus classical computer games: a randomized double-blind prospective trial of cognitive stimulation. Neuroepidemiology, 36(2), 91-99.

Roenker, D., Cissell, G., Ball, K., Wadley, V., & Edwards, J. (2003). Speed of processing and driving simulator training result in improved driving performance. Human Factors, 45: 218-233.

Shatila, E., Metzerb, A., Horvitzc, O., & Millerb, A. (2010). Home-based personalized cognitive training in MS patients: A study of adherence and cognitive performance NeuroRehabilitation 26 (2010) 143–153.

Small, G. (2005). The memory prescription: Dr. Gary Small's 14-day plan to keep your brain and body young. Hyperion.

Smith, G. E., …. Mahncke, H. W., & Zelinski, E. M. (2009). A cognitive training program based on principles of brain plasticity: Results from the Improvement in Memory with Plasticity-based Adaptive Cognitive Training (IMPACT) study. Journal of the American Geriatrics Society, 57(4), 594-603.

Stahre, L., Tärnell, B., Håkanson, C.-E., & Hällström, T. (2007). A randomized controlled trial of two weight-reducing short-term group treatment programs for obesity with an 18-month follow-up. International Journal of Behavioral Medicine, 14(1), 48-55

Tang, Y.-Y., Lu, Q., Geng, X., Stein, E. A., Yang, Y., Posner, M. I. (2010). Short-term meditation induces white matter changes in the anterior cingulate. Proceedings of the National Academy of Sciences, 107(35), 5649-15652.

Tang, Y., Ma, Y., Wang, J., Fan, Y., Feng, S., Lu, Q., et al. (2007). Short-term meditation training improves attention and self-regulation. Proceedings of the National Academy of Sciences, 104(43), 17152-17156.

Unverzagt, F. W., Guey, L. T., Jones, R. N., Marsiske, M., King, J. W., Wadley, V. G., Crowe, M., Rebok, G. W., & Tennstedt, S. L. (2012). ACTIVE Cognitive Training and Rates of Incident Dementia. J Int Neuropsychol Soc. Mar 9:1-9. [Epub ahead of print] van Leeuwen, S., Muller, N. G., & Melloni, L. (2009). Age effects on attentional blink performance in meditation. Consciousness and Cognition 18(3), 593-599.

Walton, K. G., Schneider, R. H., & Nidich, S. (2004). Review of Controlled Research on the Transcendental Meditation Program and Cardiovascular Disease: Risk Factors, Morbidity, and Mortality. Cardiology in Review, 12, 262-266.

Williams, J. W., Plassman, B. L., Burke, J., Holsinger, T., & Benjamin, S. (2010). Preventing Alzheimer's Disease and Cognitive Decline. NIH Evidence Report: AHRQ Publication.

Willis, S. L., Tennstedt, S. L., Marsiske, M., Ball, K., Elias, J., Koepke, K. M., Morris, J. N., Rebok, G. W. Unverzagt, F. W. Stoddard, A. M., & Wright, E. (2006). Long-term effects of cognitive training on everyday functional outcomes in older adults. Journal of the American Medical Association, 296(23), 2805-2814.

Wolinsky, F. D., Vander Weg, M. W., Martin, R., Unverzag, F. W., Willis, S. L., Marsiske, M., Rebok, G. W., Morris, J. N., Ball, K. K., & Tennstedt, S. L. (2010). Does Cognitive Training Improve Internal Locus of Control Among Older Adults? J Gerontol B Psychol Sci Soc Sci, 65B (5), 591-598.

Woodruff, L., & Woodruff, B. (2007). In an Instant: A Family's journey of love and healing. Random House.

Zelinski, E. M., Spina, L. M., Yaffe, K., Ruff, R., Kennison, R. F., Mahncke, H. W., & Smith, G. E. (2011). Improvement in Memory with Plasticity-Based Adaptive Cognitive Training: Results of the 3-Month Follow-Up. Journal of the American Geriatrics Society, 59(2), 258–265.

INDEX

A

accumulation of beta-amyloid protein 108

action video games 114, 248

ACTIVE study 84, 169–170, 193–195, 233

aerobic exercise 63, 75, 78, 80–83, 88, 121, 123, 200–201, 218, 221, 233, 238, 244–245

age-related decline 25, 97, 111, 195, 213, 250

alcohol consumption 93, 97, 219, 237

Alzheimer's disease 8, 10, 28, 47, 49, 54–55, 60, 66, 70, 79–80, 88, 93–95, 97–98, 108–109, 111, 116, 120, 125, 141, 208, 233, 242–243, 246–247, 249–250, 252, 255, 259

amygdala 22, 59, 125–126, 138, 145–146, 168, 188, 220, 233, 236, 250, 254

angiogenesis 76, 85

anticipation 235

antioxidants 93–94, 219

anxiety 10, 137, 146, 166, 168, 183, 185, 208, 253, 256

APOE e4 gene 55

attention 2, 10–11, 16–17, 21–22, 24, 28–29, 31, 33, 36, 38–43, 46, 57, 59, 66–67, 81, 98, 103, 107, 113–114, 123, 141–142, 144, 146, 149, 151, 159, 162–167, 170, 187, 189, 196–199, 204, 206–208, 229, 233–234, 236–237, 239, 242, 247–248, 257–258

attentional control 69, 93, 123, 145, 166–167, 246

B

BBC study 9, 54

Beck, Judith 154, 168, 184–185, 256

berries 95, 101

beta-amyloid protein 108

Bilder, Robert 56, 227

bilingualism 113, 248

biofeedback 58, 147, 155, 157, 160, 172–173, 184, 202, 205, 211, 221, 234, 237, 254–255

blood-brain barrier (BBB) 91, 219, 234

board games 112

Brain-Derived Neurotrophic Factor (BDNF) 76, 237

brain development 29–31, 66, 105

Made in the USA
Columbia, SC
16 March 2018